Game-Based Teaching and Simulation in Nursing and Healthcare

Eric B. Bauman, PhD, RN, is Associate Director for the Simulation Centers of Excellence at DeVry Inc., which includes Chamberlain College of Nursing, Carrington College, and Ross University. Dr. Bauman previously held the position of Faculty Associate at the University of Wisconsin at Madison, where he taught Crisis Management and Resuscitation, Required Clerkship in Anesthesiology, and Educational Leadership and Facilitating Learning for Adults. He also provided instruction and curricula for several nursing and other clinical departments at University of Wisconsin Hospital and Clinics. He has presented widely on Games-Based Teaching and Learning and Simulation. Dr. Bauman is currently serving as an abstract and grant reviewer for *STTI* and was a contributing editor for *Teaching and Learning in 3D Immersive Worlds*. He is also a contributing editor for *MedEdWorld* and the managing member of Clinical Playground, LLC, a company focused on Game and Simulation-Based Learning for Emergency Services and Health Sciences Education (Madison, WI). He is an Instructor/Training Center Faculty (Emergency Education Center, University of Wisconsin Hospital and Clinics), and a paramedic/firefighter. He has received several funded grants, including a GE Healthcare grant for Evaluation of Navigator Therapy in a simulator environment. He was a co-founder of the web-based portal *Games and Simulation for Healthcare* at the Ebling Health Sciences Library (University of Wisconsin – Madison). Dr. Bauman's publications include three journal articles, four book chapters, and six abstracts. He has received many honors, including Award of Gratitude, University of Wisconsin – Madison School of Nursing, and was a nominee for Dean's Teaching Award, University of Wisconsin School of Medicine and Public Health. Dr. Bauman also remains active with the Society for Simulation in Healthcare (SSH) where he serves on several committees and the International Nursing Association for Clinical Simulation and Nursing (INACSL).

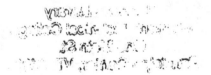

Game-Based Teaching and Simulation in Nursing and Healthcare

Eric B. Bauman, PhD, RN

SPRINGER PUBLISHING COMPANY

NEW YORK

Springer Publishing Company, LLC
11 West 42nd Street
New York, NY 10036
www.springerpub.com

Acquisitions Editor: Margaret Zuccarini
Production Editor: Michael O'Connor
Composition: Techset Composition Ltd., Salisbury, UK.

ISBN: 978-0-8261-0969-9
E-book ISBN: 978-0-8261-0970-5

12 13 14 15/ 5 4 3 2 1

The author and the publisher of this Work have made every effort to use sources believed to be reliable to provide information that is accurate and compatible with the standards generally accepted at the time of publication. Because medical science is continually advancing, our knowledge base continues to expand. Therefore, as new information becomes available, changes in procedures become necessary. We recommend that the reader always consult current research, specific institutional policies, and current drug references before performing any clinical procedure or administering any drug. The author and publisher shall not be liable for any special, consequential, or exemplary damages resulting, in whole or in part, from the readers' use of, or reliance on, the information contained in this book. The publisher has no responsibility for the persistence or accuracy of URLs for external or third-party Internet Web sites referred to in this publication and does not guarantee that any content on such Web sites is, or will remain, accurate or appropriate.

Library of Congress Cataloging-in-Publication Data
Game-based teaching and simulation in nursing and healthcare/Eric B. Bauman.
   p. ; cm.
 Includes bibliographical references and index.
 ISBN 978-0-8261-0969-9 -- ISBN 978-0-8261-0970-5
 I. Bauman, Eric B.
 [DNLM: 1. Education, Nursing--methods. 2. Clinical Medicine--education. 3. Computer
   Simulation. 4. Video Games. WY 18]
   610.73--dc23

                                                                          2012017120

Special discounts on bulk quantities of our books are available to corporations, professional associations, pharmaceutical companies, healthcare organizations, and other qualifying groups.

If you are interested in a custom book, including chapters from more than one of our titles, we can provide that service as well.

For details, please contact:
Special Sales Department, Springer Publishing Company, LLC
11 West 42nd Street, 15th Floor, New York, NY 10036-8002s
Phone: 877-687-7476 or 212-431-4370; Fax: 212-941-7842
Email: sales@springerpub.com

Printed in the United States of America Bang Printing

Throughout this book I have worked diligently to provide a collaborative multi-disciplinary approach to chapter content and expertise. To this end I would like to dedicate this book to two of my most cherished mentors, Professor Elisabeth "Betty" Hayes and Professor Emerta Mary Keller.

Contents

Contributors

Allan Barclay, MLIS, AHIP, Senior Academic Librarian & Information Architect, University of Wisconsin – Madison

Bethany Bryant, Vice President, Digitalmill, Inc

Penny Ralston-Berg, MS, Instructional Designer, Penn State World Campus

Ben DeVane, PhD, Assistant Professor, Digital Worlds Institute, University of Florida – Gainsville

Matt Gaydos, MS, Doctoral Candidate, School of Education, University of Wisconsin – Madison, and member of the Games + Learning + Society research group

Pamela Kato, PhD, EdM, Senior Research Scientist, University Medical Center Utrecht, Utrecht, Netherlands

Miguel Lara, MS, Distance Education Specialist – Instructional Consulting, School of Education, Indiana University

Renee Pyburn, MS, RN, Senior Clinical Planning Consultant, Sidra Medical & Research Center – Qatar Foundation

Gerald Stapleton, MS, Director of Distance Education, Department of Medical Education, University of Illinois at Chicago

Moses Wolfenstein, PhD, Associate Director of Research, Academic ADL CoLab, University of Wisconsin – Extension

---

Technical Editor, Mary Jo Trapani

Foreword

The complexity of today's healthcare systems demands that new graduates and professionals be prepared to care for acutely ill and complex patients in increasingly diverse settings. National leadership groups and organizations are calling for education transformation based on the *Future of Nursing Education* (IOM, 2011). Healthcare educators are now being asked to better prepare graduates to become knowledgeable workers and critical thinkers so that they can implement evidence-based interventions, and integrate emerging technologies into today's complex healthcare systems. As a result, educators are assessing the ways in which current educational programs struggle to meet the needs of healthcare professionals today. They are searching for ways to better ready students for the complexities, realities, and challenges of today's clinical practice settings. Educators are working to develop new approaches to current pedagogical methodologies that incorporate emerging technology into innovative, interprofessional, and internationally collaborative healthcare education. Foremost among new approaches are clinical simulations, virtual worlds, and interactive gaming, the topic and focus of *Game-Based Teaching and Simulation in Nursing and Healthcare*.

Clinical simulations, virtual worlds, and interactive gaming are types of pedagogies that transform the way we educate and prepare learners for clinical challenges. Simulations are a powerful strategy to engage and provide active learning with students; educators become facilitators of learning by creating interactive events and activities that reflect reality, where students can practice, acquire knowledge, and attain skills in a safe, nonthreatening environment. Simultaneously, students become active participants and controllers of their own learning when immersed in simulations, interactive gaming, or other emerging technologies.

This text has been written and disseminated at a perfect time. In answer to the call for educational transformation, healthcare education is under the microscope as its stakeholders explore best practices and methods to prepare the learners and practitioners we need today. Considering effective ways to teach today's learners, Bauman and his co-authors have developed educational strategies using emerging technologies that have the potential to redesign our clinical education. The context-rich nature of games, virtual worlds, and simulations provides examples of how nursing and other healthcare professional students can be prepared for clinical encounters and experiences. The situational models described in this book provide, controlled, and standardized environments where students can learn in an immersive manner. The authors provide an evidence-based, theoretically driven approach to implementing, integrating, and evaluating games, virtual worlds, and simulations into the curriculum for clinical education. While guiding the reader through the evolving field of virtual environments and game-based learning in nursing and healthcare, the book also discusses key elements such as curricular fit for these emerging technologies and research considerations for using them in today's educational arena. Overall, this book provides the foundation for using and integrating these emerging technologies into the learning environment, thus becoming an important faculty development plan for health professional educators wanting to incorporate these strategies into their teaching. Finally, the authors provide many resources and examples for these emerging technologies on how and where they are being used.

Game-Based Teaching and Simulation in Nursing and Healthcare is written by educators who have been immersed in this technological world exploring, testing, and evaluating these methods of instruction. The book is a valuable resource for those embarking on the use of virtual reality, game-based learning, and the use of simulations in their teaching and learning practices.

Pamela R. Jeffries PhD, RN, FAAN, ANEF
Professor and Associate Dean for Academic Affairs
Johns Hopkins University School of Nursing
Baltimore, Maryland

REFERENCE

IOM (Institute of Medicine). 2011. *The Future of Nursing: Leading Change, Advancing Health*, Washington, DC: The National Academies Press.

Preface

Game-Based Teaching and Simulation in Nursing and Healthcare provides educators with new and innovative approaches to preparing students for clinical practice and engaging nurses and other healthcare professionals in continuing education and lifelong learning. While educators now increasingly broadly adapt simulation into the curriculum, particularly mannikin-based simulation, related teaching pedagogies centered on game-based learning continue to represent less travelled and unchartered approaches to clinical education. This textbook draws from experiential learning models such as Benner's "thinking-in-action" and "novice-to-expert" (Benner, 1984) frameworks and introduces contemporary learning models specifically designed to leverage technology to engage what Prensky (2001) has termed the digital native. These contemporary theories and frameworks are specific to games and simulation and include "socially situated cognition" (Gee, 2003), "created environments" (Bauman, 2007), "designed experience" (Squire, 2006), and the ecology of culturally competent design (Bauman, 2010; Bauman and Games 2011; Games and Bauman, 2011).

Innovative technology highlighted throughout this book moves beyond standard eLearning platforms and mannikin-based simulation to include technology that until very recently has been seen as a mode for entertainment, not education. The authors of this textbook advocate using the technology of video games and virtual worlds to engage today's tech-savvy students in nursing and other clinical training programs with a host of expectations based on their sense of media literacy.

Game-Based Teaching and Simulation in Nursing and Healthcare encourages nursing scholars and educators and our colleagues across the health sciences to take a truly inter-professional perspective when approaching academic tasks such as curriculum development, implementation, and evaluation. By inter-professional we mean that various clinical disciplines ought to teach and learn together, but also that nursing and related disciplines must work in collaboration with experts in other fields who are driving the contemporary game-based learning and simulation movement. To this end, some of the brightest innovators in the fields of

educational technology, leadership, and curriculum and instruction collaborated, contributed, and co-authored various chapters and sections of
this text, to pair clinical expertise with expertise among thought leaders
in the game-based learning and simulation movement.

This text is divided into three sections. The first section focuses on
language and theories that support simulation, game-based and virtual-
world learning. The second section provides the reader with a "how-to"
guide for integrating game-based learning strategies into curricula and the
classroom. Section three offers strategies for assessing both teaching and
learning that is steeped in game-based learning encounters. In addition,
section three discusses the emerging research opportunities associated
with game-based learning methods occurring in virtual environments.
The text also offers an appendix, which includes a broad sampling of
game and simulation resources and products specific to clinical education,
as well as a glossary of terms specific to the simulation and game-based
learning literature.

Section one includes three chapters. Chapter one discusses the evolving field of virtual environments and game-based learning from a pedagogical and practical perspective. Chapter two stresses on the importance of
multi-media literacy from multiple academic perspectives. Chapter three
discusses the traditional theoretical underpinnings of contemporary pedagogy supporting the modern game-based learning movement and provides
guidance on how educators can put these theories into practice now in
their own classrooms with today's students.

Section two includes four chapters. Chapter four provides a robust discussion and road map for preparing faculty and students success when
leveraging game-based learning and virtual spaces. Chapter four details
the importance of seeking out champions, developing advocates, and
meeting stakeholder expectations. Chapter five builds on the theme of
preparation, but focuses on how the technology highlighted throughout
the text can be used to prepare learners for actual clinical environments.
Chapter six addresses the concerns and challenges associated with integrating new technology, specifically game-based learning and simulation into
existing and new curricula. Chapter seven centers on how game-based
learning and virtual environments can and should be leveraged for the
essential, but often neglected topic of cultural competency among pre-
licensure candidates and more experienced clinicians transitioning to
diverse professional roles. Even more important, chapter seven emphasizes
not only the diverse patient populations that nurses serve, but also the
increasingly diverse cultural climates that nurses and other clinicians

work in and among. This diversity emphasizes the need for innovative training opportunities that simply are not possible in traditional educational settings.

Finally, section three includes two chapters. Chapter eight centers on evaluation of both teaching and learning. When educators engage in new teaching methods it is important to evaluate these methods for effectiveness. In other words, is a game-based strategy effective in implementing curriculum objectives? And while it is always important to evaluate educators' teaching as a matter of best practice, it is essential when teachers are engaging new and innovative strategies. Chapter nine compels readers to seek out and identify research opportunities associated with game-based learning and virtual learning environments. Chapter nine provides the novice with basic concepts related to educational research and encourages all educators to become stakeholders in the research process. To accomplish this, the chapter provides examples and tips for research success based on the authors' experience.

In general, *Game-Based Teaching and Simulation in Nursing and Healthcare* provides strategies for developing, integrating, and evaluating game-based learning methods for nursing and healthcare educators. The text prepares teachers for the paradigm shift from static didactic classrooms and often asynchronous eLearning platforms to dynamic experiential learning that takes place in digital, virtual, and hybrid environments. The authors have included case studies throughout the chapters to help readers re-envision what counts for legitimate learning spaces and curricula. All of the contributors of this book urge readers to approach the material and discussion in this book with an open mind.

The aim of embracing new teaching strategies should be learner centered. Good teaching is generally not easy for the teacher, but it should be relatively easy for the learner. The vision of this book is to serve as an introduction and guide for teachers, administrators, and scholars who realize the importance of digital literacy, technology, and innovation for nursing and other clinical disciplines.

Eric B. Bauman

REFERENCES

Benner, P. (1984). *From novice to expert: Excellence and power in clinical nursing practice*. Menlo Park, CA: Addison-Wesley.

Bauman, E. (2007). High fidelity simulation in healthcare. Ph.D. dissertation, The University of Wisconsin – Madison, United States. Dissertations & Theses @ CIC Institutions database. (Publication no. AAT 3294196 ISBN: 9780549383109 ProQuest document ID: 1453230861)

Bauman, E. (2010). Virtual reality and game-based clinical education. In K. B. Gaberson, & M. H. Oermann, (Eds.), *Clinical teaching strategies in nursing education* (3rd ed). New York, Springer Publishing Company.

Bauman, E. B. & Games, I. A. (2011). Contemporary theory for immersive worlds: Addressing engagement, culture, and diversity. In A. Cheney, & R. Sanders, (Eds.), *Teaching and Learning in 3D Immersive Worlds: Pedagogical models and constructivist approaches*. IGI Global.

Games, I., & Bauman, E. (2011). Virtual worlds: An environment for cultural sensitivity education in the health sciences. *International Journal of Web Based Communities*, 7(2), 187–205.

Gee, J. P. (2003). *What videogames have to teach us about learning and literacy*. New York, NY: Palgrave-McMillan.

Prensky, M. (2001). Digital natives, digital immigrants part 1. *On the Horizon*, 9(5), 2–6.

Squire, K. (2006). From content to context: Videogames as designed experience. *Educational Researcher*, 35(8), 19–29.

Acknowledgments

In hopes of providing the reader with the best and most robust perspectives for applying game-based teaching and learning to nursing and clinical education, co-authors helped write and develop many of the chapters in this text. This book simply could not have been written without the collaboration of these colleagues.

In the spirit of multi-disciplinary and inter-professional learning I would like to say a little bit more about Professor Elisabeth "Betty" Hayes and Professor Emerta Mary Keller. Professor Hayes served as my doctoral mentor. With her encouragement I had the confidence to pursue a new field that few had heard about and even fewer understood. Professor Hayes was the inspiration for the "good game equals good simulation" epiphany that has shaped much of my scholarship. Dr. Hayes is one of the principles of the game-based learning movement and is currently a professor at Arizona State University.

Professor Keller was a member of the University of Wisconsin – Madison School of Nursing faculty from 1986 to 2006. I knew Professor Keller prior to entering graduate school; she was one of my first professors in graduate school. She taught my research methods course and provided me with encouragement through careful mentoring related to the style and effectiveness of my writing. Sadly Professor Keller succumbed to cancer in 2006 before I finished my graduate training, but not before she left a positive impact on countless nursing students and scholars.

In addition, I would like to acknowledge and thank Drs. Parvati Dev and William LeRoy Heinrich of CliniSpace™ for providing the images for the cover of this textbook. Finally, On behalf of all of the co-authors and collaborators I would like to thank Springer Publishing Company and our editor Margaret Zuccarini and her many colleagues for their patience and guidance during this adventure. Without Margaret's careful and thoughtful mentoring I am not sure this project would have ever been finished.

Game-Based Teaching and Simulation in Nursing and Healthcare

I

Language and Theory for Virtual and Game-Based Learning in Nursing and Healthcare

1

Evolving Field of Virtual Environments and Game-Based Learning in Nursing

ERIC B. BAUMAN AND MOSES WOLFENSTEIN

INTRODUCTION

*I*n this chapter the authors review the history of the use of technology in clinical education. We begin with the introduction of early mannikin-based simulation and move through a discussion of the introduction and integration of high-fidelity mannikin-based simulation. Next, the discussion will advance toward the emergence and introduction of game-based learning and virtual environments and the role that they will come to occupy in nursing and other types of clinical education. This review provides an understanding of the path taken by clinical educators to introduce and use game-based learning in virtual learning spaces specifically created to produce targeted experiences for learners.

In this chapter we introduce the reader to the importance of understanding contemporary educational theory that supports the digital shift in nursing and clinical education in general. We will explore this theory in more depth in subsequent chapters. This said, many authors of traditional educational theory and nursing theory could not have anticipated the practice environments in which nurses have come to work, nor could they have imagined the role that technology has come to play in modern learning and clinical environments. This is not to say that traditional theory no longer has a role to play in nursing and other types of clinical education. It has never been appropriate for clinical educators to design curricula based only on tradition or historical practice. Rather, we argue in this text that understanding stakeholder expectations helps educational designers and teachers glean valuable lessons from past practice while they embrace contemporary educational theory that supports and even anticipates future clinical practice that represents the digital shift in educational practice.

3

In this chapter and throughout this text we stress the importance of ensuring that curriculum objectives drive game-based digital environments designed for learning, in this case clinical nursing education. Using technology for the sake of technology can confuse and frustrate students, teaching faculty, and staff. Not all course objectives are best addressed by using new or emerging technology. Selecting course objectives that leverage and provide a good fit for game-based learning is essential to ensuring the success of strategies for instruction that rely on multimedia environments.

HISTORY OF EMERGING TECHNOLOGY IN CLINICAL EDUCATION

Traditionally, educators have taught nursing and other health sciences disciplines by using familiar methods that saturate the early part of the curriculum with often redundant and repetitive didactic content from one course to another (Giddens & Brady, 2007). Teachers then slowly introduce students to hands-on clinical experiences. As students demonstrate a mastery of didactic content through traditional examination, teachers, clinical instructors, and faculty allow students to participate in more complex clinical encounters. The hope is that the students' mastery of traditional didactic content will provide a translational context for increasingly complex clinical environments. To a large extent this process represents an apprentice style of education (Allan, 2010; Merriam & Caffarella, 2007).

Over the last decade, nursing and other clinical health sciences have begun to embrace and leverage technology to provide situated learning experiences. These experiences draw from previous and concurrent didactic lessons that help prepare students for new clinical environments and encounters. Simulation-based (SB) technology, specifically SB learning using high-fidelity mannikins is now commonplace in many undergraduate nursing programs (Shinnick, Woo, & Mentes, 2011). This said, historically various professions have employed SB learning in general to prepare students for professional practices that involve high-risk encounters that occur infrequently (DeVita, 2005; Gaba, Howard, Fish, Smith, & Sowb, 2001; Helmreich, 2000). Examples of industries on the forefront of SB learning include commercial aviation, maritime and commercial shipping, nuclear power production, and many aspects of military training (Bauman, 2007; Gaba, 2004; Schaefer & Grenvik, 2001; Shapiro & Simmons, 2002; Ziv, Wolpe, Small, & Glick, 2003). These industries continue to provide leadership in SB learning.

In healthcare, disciplines that routinely involve the management of complex, high-risk patient care settings have embraced SB learning, including trauma resuscitation, cardiac resuscitation, and anesthesia crisis management (Gaba, 2004; Lee et al., 2003; McLellan, 1999). While the introduction of high-fidelity SB instruction in the health sciences initially focused on high-risk, low-incidence event training, it is now being used much more broadly as the literature supporting SB education has grown (Campbell & Daley, 2009). This is not to say that healthcare disciplines do not use various types of simulation, but rather educators now apply more complex technology to SB learning taking place within the context of nursing and other types of clinical education.

Teachers have employed low-fidelity simulation to introduce nursing students to the fundamentals of nursing care for many years. In fact, teachers have used mannikins for various forms of simple simulation in healthcare training for centuries. Ziv et al. (2003) discussed the role of early simulation dating back to the 16th century when "phantoms," a type of simple mannikin, served as proxies for actual patients during obstetrical training and practice (Bauman, 2007). The contemporary beginnings of mannikin-based instruction in healthcare began with the introduction of Cardio Pulmonary Resuscitation (CPR) training. In 1961, several anesthesiologists tasked Asmund Laerdal, a Norwegian toy manufacturer, with creating a realistic mannikin suitable for teaching the technique of mouth-to-mouth ventilation. Shortly after Asmund Laerdal's initial airway mannikin inception, Laerdal enhanced the airway mannikin to include an external cardiac massage component (chest compressions). This simulator, known as the Resusci-Anne® and others like it continue to be used today to train thousands in CPR. The Laerdal Company now manufactures many medical devices, a host of comprehensive and complex patient simulators, including the SimMan® 3G (Grenvik & Schaefer, 2004). In the last 10 years the number of manufacturers making and distributing simulators designed specifically for nursing and health sciences education has grown exponentially. More recently, Laerdal has embraced the paradigm shift toward multimedia and online learning by producing distributive learning modules for a variety of clinicians.

While Resusci-Anne® was being developed in Europe, other mannikin-based simulators began to emerge in the United States, including the Sim1 (Cooper & Taqueti, 2004; Lane, Slavin, & Ziv, 2001; Tan, Ti, Suresh, Ho, & Lee, 2002). Stephan Abrahamson, an engineer, developed Sim1 with physician Judson Denson in the mid-1960s. Cooper and Taqueti (2004) called Sim1 the "starting point for true computer-controlled mannikin simulators, particularly for simulation of the entire patient" (p. 112). The advantage of the Sim1 and other simulators like it was that it provided a platform for teaching specific tasks, including endotracheal intubation, an advanced airway skill. This allowed potentially dangerous skills like endotracheal intubation, which is an invasive procedure, to be taught in a manner that eliminated risk to patients. Basic proficiency could be taught, mastered, and evaluated through simulation allowing novices to become proficient prior to attempting the procedure on an actual patient (Gordon, Oriol, & Cooper, 2004). Medical Education Technologies, Incorporated (METI) of Sarasota, Florida (now CAE Healthcare, a Canadian company) eventually developed a full-scale, comprehensive, complex mannikin, that combines various aspects of task or procedural training with dynamic human patient physiology software capable of modeling numerous patient conditions, pathologies, and related treatment modalities.

Substantial information sharing between health sciences and engineering disciplines related to SB education is a relatively new phenomenon. The jump from the rather simple Resusci-Anne®-style simulator to the modern, more comprehensive simulator capable of modeling human physiology took place within the high-acuity field of anesthesiology, and to a lesser extent, cardiology (Cooper & Taqueti, 2004; Hammond, Bermann, Chen, & Kushins, 2002; Howard et al., 2003; Kneebone, 2005).

Physician Michael Gordon developed a simulator known as "Harvey" in the 1960s and first demonstrated it in 1968. Gordon designed Harvey, named after Gordan's mentor, W. Proctor Harvey, to simulate various cardiac conditions to develop students' cardiac diagnostic abilities. The Harvey simulator also provided a standardized comprehensive platform for evaluating students (Cooper & Taqueti, 2004). The ability for instructors to introduce a standard platform that can be consistently integrated into curricula over time is one of the hallmarks of the SB learning movement. Standardization affords all students the same educational experiences in preparation for independent clinical practice.

In the 1980s, innovators developed several other anesthesia-specific simulators and introduced them into health sciences education. David Gaba, a Stanford Medical School physician, developed the Comprehensive Anesthesia Simulation Environment (CASE). He designed the CASE system less as a mechanism for honing clinical assessment or task-specific skills like intubation or airway management, and more as a system for evaluating the human response to critical events in terms of performance assessment and behavioral response (Gaba, 2004). Physician Michael Good and J.S. Gravenstein, an engineer at the University of Florida, were also developing the Gainsville Anesthesia Simulator (GAS) in the 1980s. Unlike Resusci-Anne® and Harvey, the anesthesia-specific simulators were designed not as task trainers, but as mechanisms to increase patient safety and positively affect patient outcome before, during, and after students' training (Bauman, 2007; Cooper & Taqueti, 2004).

The shift from using simulators to teach and evaluate specific tasks to be mastered by students, to using simulators as the stage or platform for designing, implementing, and evaluating behavioral change demonstrates the important shift in how technology can become integrated into existing curricula. We might consider leveraging virtual simulation that takes place in game-based or virtual environments in the same way we have in the now familiar mannikin-based simulation laboratory. The mannikin-based simulator must exist in a fixed location, a laboratory or *in situ*, and is often only accessible to students based on schedules that are designed around institutions' business hours. Further, even a modest single mannikin simulation laboratory can cost well over $100,000 in initial capital costs alone. Game-based learning environments existing in digital or virtual reality environments literally play by a different set of rules. Virtual environments do occupy space, but in a very different context that challenges the conventional notions of time and real estate.

THE DIGITAL SHIFT: FROM THE CLASSROOM TO THE SIMULATION LAB ON THE WAY TO VIRTUAL OR GAME-BASED ENVIRONMENTS

Educators can and should harness new methods of instruction that use technology to prepare nursing students and other health sciences students for those experiences that cannot be guaranteed during traditional didactic and clinical methods of education. As the role of the registered nurse continues to grow in terms of clinical complexity and professional and personal liability, it becomes more challenging but evermore important to prepare new graduates for the types of complex patients and environments they will encounter in actual practice. Unfortunately, traditional modalities of nursing education cannot consistently guarantee exposure to all of the relevant clinical educational opportunities needed to prepare students and later new graduates for the transition from novice to expert (Benner, 1984; Benner, Tanner, & Chesla, 2009; Larew, Lessans, Spunt, Foster, & Covington, 2006).

This is not to imply that graduating students should enter their professions as experts, but instead to imply that new graduates and novice clinicians must be able to enter their professions with valuable experiences to build on as they attain clinical expertise (Benner et al., 2009). Clinical encounters of educational value need not be left to chance; these situations can be designed through simulation and game-based learning to ensure that all students have the opportunity to experience consistent curricula and comprehensive instruction (Bauman, 2010; Bauman & Games, 2011; Friedrich, 2002; Games & Bauman, 2011; Gordon et al., 2004; Lane et al., 2001; Shapiro & Simmons, 2002; Ziv et al., 2003).

The traditional nursing laboratory provides learners with a physical space to engage in the many tasks of nursing in a safe environment, without risk of negative consequence to patients while attending to the relative emotional safety of the learner. In the traditional nursing laboratory, students are introduced to skills such as bed making, bathing, wound care, sterile technique, and later more complex skills such as patient interviewing and assessment. Traditional nursing skills laboratories generally include a number of low-fidelity mannikins that allow students to learn and later be evaluated on any number of skills associated with nursing practice. These traditional laboratories continue to play an important role in nursing education. Adding high-fidelity simulators and game-based learning environments into the curriculum simply because they are available often leaves learners confused and teachers frustrated. Exploring and understanding where and when to leverage this technology is essential to successfully integrate the technology into the curriculum.

For example, using a $100,000 mannikin simulator to teach students how to change linens with a patient in the bed is a poor and expensive proxy for a simple low-fidelity mannikin or a standardized patient who could very well be role-played by another student. Similarly, students will not glean any *haptic* feedback from starting an IV or completing a blood draw in a digital game-based virtual environment.

Instead, educators should see game-based learning as an integrative step toward supervised clinical practice and eventual independent clinical practice. Game-based learning in virtual environments should also be seen as a step toward actual practice, just as SB learning in a fixed or created space serves as an integrated step toward practice in actual clinical environments (Bauman, 2007; Bauman, 2010; Bauman & Games, 2011; Games & Bauman, 2011).

Mannikin-based simulation acts as an intermediate step between didactic preparation and the actual clinical environment. It allows students to perform in a created environment (Bauman, 2007; Bauman, 2010; Bauman & Games, 2011; Games & Bauman, 2011) complete with specifically designed experiences (Squire, 2006) that have been engineered to provide meaningful encounters that prepare students for actual clinical environments. A schematic of this process is found Figure 1.1.

The *Simulation to Practice Pathway* initially served as a mechanism to illustrate how teachers could integrate mannikin-based simulation into their existing curriculum (Bauman, 2007). While this process was never meant to be entirely linear, it provided a starting point for a "how-to" discussion for those interested in embracing mannikin-based simulation as a method for clinical education. In this pathway students must be prepared for the SB experience. From this perspective, including simulation in the curriculum does not

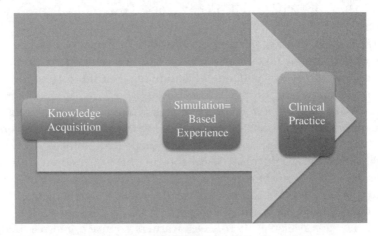

FIGURE 1.1
Simulation to practice pathway. Copyright Bauman (2007).

obviate the need for basic knowledge acquisition. This preparation, or knowledge acquisition can take place through traditional didactic pedagogical approaches. In fact, a traditional didactic approach is often the most appropriate and sensible approach given the audience and constraints associated with clinical education.

The principles of andragogy support adult learners as self-motivated students who are able and willing to take responsibility for many aspects of their educations (Merriam & Caffarela, 2007). Students who enter SB learning environments without adequate orientation to these environments and the situated content teachers reinforce often find their experiences to be confusing and frustrating. Orientation is an important facet of any learning experience. Students who are unfamiliar with the advantages and limitations of virtual spaces will require a tutorial or an orientation phase to the new virtual learning environment medium. Teachers familiar with virtual worlds sometimes refer to this phase as a *walk through*. The *walk through* provides learners with the opportunity to explore *in-world* environments with or without an active tutorial. Just as it is important for students to be adequately prepared for supervised clinical environments, it is also important for them to be prepared for situated learning experiences that leverage SB learning in fixed laboratories or in virtual environments (Bauman, 2007).

When done well, particularly during initial training, the simulation laboratory provides an important place for instructors to test the waters with their students who may be operating at the edge of their knowledge base in a safe environment that provides experiences specifically designed to support later learning and actual practice (Bauman, 2007; Squire, 2006). As we embrace the digital shift in higher education, how we define the clinical laboratory and simulation laboratory will shift from fixed, created spaces to include virtual and online spaces often encompassing game-based learning scenarios.

As educators continue to recognize games, *serious games*, and game-based learning as legitimate pedagogical tools in kindergarten through high school education, and in higher education, including professional, clinical, and technical education, it becomes necessary to examine how and where educators can best leverage games to enhance student experiences that provide translational utility. The inclusion of games in the curriculum must aid the learning experience not only from the aesthetic perspective, but also through the ability to better prepare students for actual clinical practice. From this perspective we are not arguing that games and game-based learning should replace SB learning found in fixed spaces or that they somehow replace the didactic component of clinical education. Rather, we argue that educators can and should see game-based learning as an available resource to engage students in meaningful experiences that inform both their educational experience and future clinical practice. The rethought simulation to practice pathway below demonstrates the role that game-based learning should play during clinical education and is shown in Figure 1.2 (Bauman, 2010).

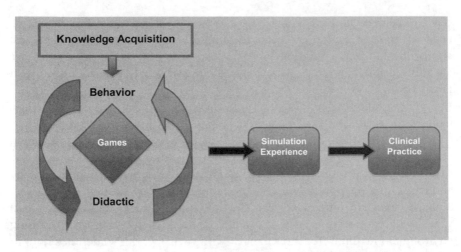

FIGURE 1.2
Rethought simulation to practice pathway. Copyright Bauman (2010).

The *Rethought Simulation to Practice Pathway* incorporates games as an integrated process beginning at the knowledge aquisition level. Game-based learning in this model begins as an integrated component of learner knowledge aquistion. Again, the model is not meant to be linear. Nor should educators see the integration of games into curriculum as an opportunity to be engaged only at the beginning of a learning process or curriculum. Also note that when educators integrate game-based learning into the traditional didactic phase of clinical education, they provide an active behavioral component that situates learner expereince. Adding the *behavioral* facet as an accompanying component to the *knowledge acquisition* phase of this model is quite deliberate.

Traditional forms of didactic presentation are content oriented. They are static and do not engage learners through interaction based on narrative, decision making, and consequence. This is not to say that traditional didactic content cannot include narrative components. Instead games have the potential to engage learners differently than traditional aspects of didactic presentation, such as reading assignments or lectures.

Addressing behavioral expectations associated with the clinical environment is very difficult to do in the traditional didactic component of nursing and other clinical sciences disciplines. Static content simply cannot model behavior and introduce the social and professional mores associated with professional practice in the same way that an interactive game-based environment can. Further, the interactive game-based environment allows students to test their knowledge in a venue that is contextually situated in terms of patient and professional consequences related to decision making. Asking students to think about how their personal presentation, interpersonal communication style, and decision making might affect future practice and encourage students to reflect but does not necessarily engage them. An interactive game-based environment provides students with an experience specifically engineered to introduce students to specific targeted objectives (Squire, 2006). Moreover, sharing an experience together, perhaps in a virtual world, is a more powerful reflective experience than talking about similar experiences that learners have experienced independently elsewhere (Tyczkowski, Bauman, Gallagher-Lepak, Vandenhouten, & Resop Reilly, 2012).

The digital shift in nursing and clinical education is occurring throughout curriculum. As discussed above, digital educational interventions are changing the way we present basic or introductory information to novice students. Many teachers have come to equate digital leaning with online course work. However, while online courses have made great strides in terms of addressing the challenges of time and location, they often fail to engage students any more than a traditional lecture style course. In fact, some have argued that online course work that is not carefully designed to specially include student interaction is often even less engaging than traditional classroom learning (Browning, 1999; Sharpe & Hawkins, 1998).

WHY IT IS ESSENTIAL TO UNDERSTAND THEORY THAT EMBRACES THE DIGITAL SHIFT

While emerging digital learning technologies have begun to transform teaching and learning in healthcare simply as a result of their growing popularity in clinical education settings, it is essential for teachers and faculty who use them to understand the theoretical models that have given rise to these tools so that they can deploy them effectively. Digital simulation and game-based technologies have both grown up alongside a number of learning theories and stimulated the development of new theories in a variety of fields. While Chapter 3 of this book will look at game-based theories in greater depth, this chapter offers an introduction to a few of the more prominent theories tied to digital media and learning: constructionism, socially situated approaches to cognition, and the theory of designed experience. All three theoretical orientations tie in the idea that learning is best supported through interaction, and hence essential when designing, integrating, and evaluating both simulations and games.

The theory of constructionism developed by Seymour Papert is a direct descendant of the much more widely known theory of constructivism developed by Jean Piaget. While constructivism substantially predates digital technology, constructionism retains a number of its core features while translating them into a more contemporary context where digital media plays a central role. Both constructionism and constructivism share an emphasis on knowledge that is constructed by the learner rather than transmitted by the teacher. For Piaget, this was a move against the prevalent assumption that knowledge was external to the mind, a key feature of the "transmission model" of learning then in vogue. For Papert, it involved both elements of constructivist theory, and a desire to "push back" on persistent education policy initiatives that focused on improving the quality of teaching rather than the quality of learning (Papert, 1980).

Ultimately, Papert's constructionism is a pragmatic instructional theory, while constructivism (Piaget) is both cognitive and philosophical in nature. However, at their core both focus on knowledge building through experiences. Papert and Harel (1991) described the relationship between the two theories by noting that they share a "connotation of learning as 'building knowledge structures' irrespective of the circumstances of the learning" (p. 1). However, for Papert, the ultimate aim of advancing constructionism was not so much to understand learning in the capacity of development, but to reframe how we approach learning with a renewed emphasis on the making of things as the most essential aspect of real learning.

In the context of simulation and game-based learning, Papert's explicit emphasis on learning through building something may seem less applicable at first blush. However, it's worth noting that Papert developed construction-ism primarily around mathematics where displays of student learning have been traditionally limited to decontextualized or un-situated performance via paper and pencil testing. The development of constructionism can be seen in part as a way of emphasizing that as computers are brought into learning experiences, they should not be used to replace instructors, but to create opportunities for students to learn by doing (Papert, 1980). In the context of using simulation and games to prepare students for clinical encounters, con-structionism serves as a reminder that simply requiring students to use these technologies may be necessary but not sufficient to create deep learning oppor-tunities. Instead, teachers need to provide students with chances to rearticu-late their experiences of learning with digital media and engage in authentic discourse with peers and mentors regarding the learning activities they encountered in the digital environment.

While constructionism draws from Piaget's theory of constructivism, many researchers who have theorized on cognition as a socially situated pheno-menon draw on Lev Vygotsky's similarly named theory of social constructivism (Vygotsky, 1978). The core element of social constructivism that learning takes place through a complex array of social and cultural interactions is reflected in a number of learning theories and mobilized in work related to game and SB learning. In addition to technical artifacts like mannikins and curricula, the term also refers to social and cultural artifacts such as symbols and systems of organization (such as numbering systems and languages). Nursing and other clinical sciences are rich with both technical and cultural artifacts. New students often struggle with the language and system of organization inherent to nursing practice as they learn how to communicate using new terms and systems of diagnosis that are essential to competent practice.

The core tenets of social constructivism have fueled a great deal of thinking around how digital media artifacts function within learning systems. Social
constructivism highlights not only the ways in which game and simulation
tools remediate learning for individuals, but also the different ways in which
educators can leverage these tools in various social and cultural contexts.
Vygotsky's theory of social constructivism also pushes instructional designers,
teachers, and researchers to think about the relationship between the development and use of situated social and cultural artifacts found within the
digital environment.

The basic concept that learning is best understood by looking at interactions between both humans and nonhumans, in this case technology, is
taken up time and again by learning theorists who have defined the field of
digital media and learning, like John Sealy Brown (Brown & Duguid, 2001)
and James Paul Gee (Gee, 2003). Researchers Jean Lave and Etienne Wenger,
whose concept of communities of practice (Lave & Wenger, 1991) have also
greatly influenced the development and study of various digital media forms
for learning. The common thread among these researchers and their theories
is that they stem from the fundamental enterprise of viewing learning as a
socially situated activity.

James Paul Gee's *What Video Games Have to Teach Us About Learning
and Literacy* (2003) is arguably the most seminal work in the study of video
games and learning. In this work, Gee points to both the manner in which
games function as well-ordered problem spaces, and the manner in which
player communities enable powerful learning experiences (2003). In the
context of schools, Gee has subsequently emphasized that games are hardly
a universal remedy, and that he is not actually advancing an agenda around
games and learning per se. Comparatively, games offer us representations of
what he calls "situated and embodied learning." Gee explains this concept as
"being able to solve problems with what you know. Not just knowing a
bunch of inert facts, but being able to use facts and information as tools for
problem solving in specific contexts." (Brown, 2011).

Similarly Brown, Collins, and Duguid proposed the concept of "cognitive
apprenticeship" as a means of conveying the manner in which learning is inherently situated within specific sociocultural contexts that inform possible applications of knowledge (1989). Both Brown and Collins have subsequently
written separately in great depth around the topic of learning and digital
media (Collins & Halverson, 2009; Thomas & Brown, 2011). However, even
prior to the rise of these authors' perspectives on media and learning they
advanced a fundamental theory with extensive implications for using digital
games and simulation for learning. These authors noted that, "... people
who use tools actively rather than just acquire them, by contrast, build an
increasingly rich implicit understanding of the world in which they use the
tools and of the tools themselves" (Brown et al., 1989, p. 33). This notion
clearly reflects the same approach Gee adopts in pointing to the difference

between situated understandings and the acquisition of inert facts or un-situated didactic content. Brown et al. go on to note that, "Learning how to use a tool involves far more than can be accounted for in any set of explicit rules. The occasions and conditions for use arise directly out of the context of activities of each community that uses the tool, framed by the way the members of that community see the world." (p. 33).

Brown, et al. have presented an important insight into what it means for cognition to be socially situated, and one that clearly illustrates the implications of learning theory in the development and integration of game and simulation technologies. Learning is not only bound to specific contexts, as has been illustrated extensively through the literature on knowledge transfer (Bransford & Schwartz, 1999), but the application of learning is bound in cultural norms and via individual's understanding of said culture as well. In terms of the design of digital tools for learning in clinical disciplines such as nursing, this means ensuring that the representation of nursing practice includes an adequate representation of context in order for the learner to not only understand technical and nontechnical aspects of the nursing practice, but also to know when and how it is appropriate to implement those various approaches and procedures. Successful implementation of media-based technology, including game-based learning into the curriculum must emphasize the socially situated nature of cognition and how it serves as a reminder that where and at what point technology-based media tools are integrated into the learning process can be crucial in ensuring their efficacy.

Before games and simulation saw widespread use in educational settings, theorists were already advancing frameworks that have helped us make sense of how digital resources work to restructure human cognition and learning. While some of the previously enumerated 20th-century theories centered on the sociocultural and psychological aspects of learning in general, they would later be adapted to provide the pedagogical underpinnings for incorporating games and simulation into educational settings. However, even before theorists began focusing on the situated sociocultural aspects of learning, the importance of educational design and its relationship with learner experience was being explored. As early as the 19th century, Friedrich Froebel, while creating the system of kindergarten, defined early childhood education through the development of a carefully crafted series of designed interactive "gifts" (Brosterman, 1997). The moniker "kindergarten" for preelementary education would of course stick, even as the details of Froebel's carefully designed educational experience would fall away in favor of more generic learning structures. However, the concept of designing learning opportunities would be taken up again by a number of other learning theorists between the 19th century and the present day.

Chapter 3 explores the development of theories that look at the development of learning spaces as a design activity in much greater depth. For the purposes of gaining a basic orientation to digital learning resources as designed or created spaces (Bauman, 2007) in this introductory chapter, we will consider recent work by Kurt Squire which looks specifically at video games as designed experiences. While Squire's theory of games as designed experiences departs from the same socially situated assumption that other scholars have pointed to, he goes on to interpret how it is that video game designers work to create powerful learning experiences even in those games that have been designed primarily for entertainment (Squire, 2006).

Squire specifically notes that a game "... provides a set of experiences, with the assumption being that learners are active constructors of meaning with their own drives, goals, and motivations. Most good games afford multiple trajectories of participation and meaning making. Content is delivered just-in-time and on demand to solve problems" (Squire, 2006, pp. 24–25). Here Squire points to three distinct traits of high-quality video games as designed experiences that make them particularly effective for certain types of learning. He emphasizes the manner in which good game design sets up conditions for the learner to drive their own learning through the creation of meaningful goals. He emphasizes the fact that most good games provide more than one route toward mastery, thus allowing different learners a variety of ways to approach the task. Finally, he emphasizes a point that has also been highlighted by Gee (2003), that scholars concerned with assessment have since recognized as an essential feature of games for learning (Shute, 2011): games deliver new content in the support of specific contexts "just-in-time and on demand" in order to help players solve problems.

In the context of nursing education and other clinical learning, Squire's theory of games as designed experiences (and other design-centered theories of learning) have obvious import. In analyzing possible simulation and game-based learning technologies, those engaged with curricular and program development would do well to keep an eye on what the design of the artifact conveys about the assumptions of the designers, and whether or not there is a good match between the tool and learning objectives. Specifically, educators can evaluate digital learning tools based on the degree to which the game or simulation guides the learner. They can accomplish this by setting up internally consistent goals in the learning experience that map effectively onto real practice. When appropriate, such tools should also seek to provide for the variance found in real practice. When evaluating a game or simulation for clinical training learning objectives, it is essential to ensure that the feedback cycles the tool engenders are meaningful, and triggered at appropriate times to advance understanding effectively.

THE ROLE OF OBJECTIVE-BASED CURRICULA IN THE DIGITAL ENVIRONMENT

For some, the excitement of embracing new technology can overshadow existing valid and meaningful curriculum objectives. For others, embracing any change, let alone change that may require the acquisition of new skills and personal time investment related to the multimedia digital shift occurring in the clinical sciences is daunting if not intimidating. This said, occasionally, teaching institutions find self-proclaimed digital gurus and pioneers within their ranks. However, the key to leveraging the digital environment is to remember that good educational design principles start with objectives and theory. Designing curricula is much like designing a research project. All of the elements of the experiment or in this case curriculum must be present, including the course objectives. To extend the metaphor, the digital environment represents part of the methods section, but not the research question.

A common error that occurs during the introduction of digital tools involves forgetting the basic practice of aligning curricular content with learning objectives. This error also occurs when introducing game-based learning strategies into any curriculum and often results in the adoption of new technologies that may not align with or support the actual learning outcomes a program seeks to achieve. Failure to match technology to curriculum objectives or a haphazard adoption of technology-based resources without effective curricular integration and support can result in a combination of failures that may lead to a "Christmas tree" phenomenon (Bryk et al., 1998). This phenomenon can occur when a school or program continually adopts new conflicting educational technologies without effective integration, which in turn leads to a muddled learning experience. The adoption of learning technologies based on trends found in the current marketplace can lead to an accumulation of expensive unused resources. All of these issues can be effectively managed through an objective-based approach to developing a curriculum that leverages digital environments.

EXAMPLES AND CASE STUDIES OF GAME-BASED LEARNING

When recruiting digital tools for clinical education it is important to ensure that tool adoption (in this case games) is being driven by efforts to fill curricular holes, improve identified shortcomings, or generally improve the clinical experience so that students are better prepared for actual real-world practice environments. Teachers can see both successes and failures in this regard when adopting virtual worlds like *Second Life* into the clinical curriculum. Successes are marked by attempts to use these virtual worlds to rethink the failures of more traditional simulation technologies. Failures are evident in the array of now largely vacant training areas developed in these virtual worlds without consideration for how they will be used after their creation.

Various educational institutions have created virtual in-world environments within spaces like *Second Life*. However, few of those environments move beyond aesthetic appeal. By this we mean that the environments offer little more than a visually pleasing and accurate representation of an actual space like a hospital or operating room. Due to an environment void of inter-action and narrative, these spaces offer little if anything to promote curriculum objectives or translational facets of clinical education.

The New World Clinic is a *Second Life* island, created and operated by Gerald Stapleton from the University of Illinois at Chicago that moves beyond aesthetic appeal to promote specific curriculum objectives centered on patient communication and history-taking skills. Stapleton uses the New World Clinic as a virtual standardized patient laboratory. Students, through use of "avatars," interact with other in-world "players" played by trained, standardized patients.

The SimQuest game *Blast* provides civilian and military care providers with an SB game targeted at training for effective scene and patient manage-ment following explosive blast incidents. The central objective of this game is to teach the concepts of triage. The game offers an aesthetically relevant environment, but more importantly it stresses patient and environmental fide-lity. Players encounter nonplayer characters among the injured who have authentic physiology that is accurately mapped to injury and pathology. In this way, decisions that player/learners make in the environment drive outcome and consequence.

It is also worth noting that while many of the specialized digital resources designed for clinical programs can be costly, in some instances educators can repurpose less expensive tools developed outside of the clinical context or created under open source or open content licensing that may be available for nursing education. As with any other digital media, educators should accom-pany the media with an analysis of the specific learning objectives when adopt-ing or repurposing existing tools. The analysis should include the specific learning objectives that the tool can help meet, as well as a thorough consider-ation of what additional costs or requirements accompany adoption of the tool in terms of curricular and technical support.

Game and simulation development can be very costly. *Zero Hour: America's Medic* offers one example of how working collaboratively can minimize the infrastructural cost yet make good use of existing software development resources. This approach demonstrates how collaboration allows educators and content experts to focus on meaningful game content and game play to ensure that learning objectives are well mapped into the gaming experience. To develop *Zero Hour: America's Medic*, a game-based environment for preparing EMTs/Paramedics for mass casualty events, the National Emergency Medical Services Preparedness Initiative at George Washington University and Virtual Heroes/ARA, the creators of the well-known military training and recruitment game America's Army, collaborated. While creation of *Zero Hour: America's Medic* required developers to create new content and new game resources, by working with an established vendor George Washington University was able to take advantage of Virtual Heroes/ARA experience with and ability to use the *Unreal 3.0* game engine. In addition, this partnership streamlined various aspects of the project including costly licensing considerations often associated with game platform choice.

The development landscape for creating games and simulations continues to evolve. As time goes on there will be a greater diversity of tools that enable game development to take place with less programming expertise. Adobe's Dreamweaver software, and now various simplified content management systems have enabled huge numbers of users to develop websites without having a deep knowledge of HTML tags or similar programming software. Similarly, new tools now exist specifically for game development with less programming expertise on the part of the designer. The Unity software suite from Unity Technologies in San Francisco provides a particularly powerful example of a tool that allows developers and designers to create games and game-like tools with more moderate programming capacity, and at a substantially lower cost than that traditionally associated with licensing a game engine, such as *Unreal 3.0*. Similarly, Google's App Inventor allows individuals with minimal technical expertise to develop simple applications for the Android operating system.

However, the availability of middleware tools like Unity or Google App Inventor does not guarantee the quality of the product (game or simulation) that developers can create. Dreamweaver made web design more accessible, but did not necessarily increase the quality of websites. Rather it ensured that more individuals with less training in graphic design and web-based technology could create websites. Similarly, as the availability of contemporary tools for game and simulation creation increases, the potential result may be the preponderance of products yielding poor learning experiences. Creating the sort of sophisticated representations of practice that can make a digital object into a powerful learning tool ultimately requires knowledge of how the system works that one is attempting to model. However, making such models into effective game-based learning tools also requires developers and educators to understand interaction design, have specific knowledge of what makes a simulation or game effective as a learning aid, and have an awareness of the role that the instructor will ultimately play in the virtual learning space. Further, one must come to accept that the requirements for making a successful learning game existing in a virtual environment, while similar to lab-based simulation experiences, are not identical.

REUSE AND REPURPOSING

Beyond the development of new digital tools, educators can glean examples of technology reuse or repurposing from other sorts of professional preparation programs. For instance, educational leadership professor Richard Halverson (University of Wisconsin–Madison) has done extensive work in developing game and simulation-based learning solutions for in-service and preservice education leadership professionals. These efforts include Halverson's adaptation of an early open-sourced version of the code for transcription software Transana. His purpose was to develop a simple tool for helping educational professionals develop an eye for evaluating classroom teaching and learning (Halverson & Wolfenstein, 2007). In addition, Halverson has repurposed the Microsoft PowerPoint presentation software as a means to engage students with case-based learning in a more meaningful manner (Halverson, Blakesley, & Figueiredo-Brown, 2011).

The latter example offers a particularly powerful example of developing a low-cost solution to a persistent educational problem: the propensity for learners to "arm-chair" the decision making process in case-based learning interactions, rather than confront the complexity that accompanies decision making in practice. By using PowerPoint, Halverson and his team were able to focus students' attention on a new approach to case-based learning, rather than spending valuable instructional time introducing a new software tool.

Requiring nursing students to take part in the use of novel media or unfamiliar activities like game-based learning can be a challenge that often requires teachers to introduce and orient related technologies into the learning environment, whether students are undergraduates, new graduates, or advanced graduate-level learners who are used to traditional didactic instruction. For those instructors comfortable with the modern simulation lab, this is familiar territory. Orientating students so that they have an understanding of the possibilities and limitations of created environments is essential for learner success, whether they exist in virtual or physical spaces. Regardless of monetary cost, technology that is perceived as novel, new, or out of the ordinary is more likely to gain stakeholder consensus for integration into new and existing curricula when it is well understood by both teachers and students (Bauman, 2010).

Finally, educators can sometimes find powerful applications in off-the-shelf products developed for noneducational purposes. Professor Kurt Squire's (University of Wisconsin–Madison) research on the use of Sid Meier's *Civilization III*, a strategy-based video game based on and also steeped in contextually situated historical lessons stands out as a good example of how a professor effectively repurposed a product that was originally developed for entertainment purposes to teach a specific type of understanding within an educational domain (Squire, DeVane, & Durga, 2008; Squire 2011). While Squire's work describes an example of repurposing game content related to general education, it is possible to imagine examples that could relate to nursing education. Many facets of nursing education focus on communication, prioritization, and critical decision making. Some refer to these as "soft" skills, but are more appropriately termed behavioral or nontechnical skills. While modeling these types of interactions is complex, there is a growing array of commercial games designed for entertainment purposes that seek to include some of these same critical elements as part of their successful game design (e.g., BioWare's *Mass Effect* games). In addition, certain types of multiplayer games already on the market provide opportunities for players to develop these same critical skills through interaction with each other around collaborative objectives (Wolfenstein, 2010).

One thought-provoking and interesting example of entertainment-based gaming repurposed for use by the clinical sciences comes from the intersection of epidemiological research and the genre of Massively Multiplayer Online Games (MMOGs). In 2005, an unplanned event occurred in the MMOG *World of Warcraft* that provided an unparalleled research opportunity for epidemiologists to examine a population encountering an epidemic. Based on an exploit discovered by high-level players in the game, a virtual "virus" was unleashed on a large population of *player characters* in the game. Following up on a lead from her former student Eric Lofgren, epidemiologist Nina Fefferman took advantage of the opportunity to observe how the player population responded both to the virtual outbreak, and to the range of countermeasures that Blizzard, the creators of *World of Warcraft*, attempted to impose in an effort to curb the effects of the virtual epidemic (Lofgren & Fefferman, 2007). While this unplanned event presented a research rather than teaching opportunity, it provides a clear example of how a system designed for entertainment was capable of providing powerful insights with long-term implications for healthcare practices.

A somewhat more practical example of repurposing comes from studies that have looked at video games as tools to help enhance surgical training. A number of studies have focused on this topic, and a much larger range of research has been devoted to understanding what, if any, psychomotor benefits games might have for the people that play them. In a literature review of studies looking specifically at surgical ability, Lynch, Aughwane, and Hammond (2010) determined that game players seem to acquire endoscopic techniques more quickly. While further research in this area is necessary to determine the efficacy of repurposing commercial games for clinical education, the examples provided here warrant the continued evaluation of commercially available entertainment games for eventual reuse for clinical education.

SUMMARY

When instructors implement tools or resources, like digital games and simulation existing in fixed or virtual-created environments, they have the capacity to fundamentally advance the quality and depth of the educational experiences an institution offers. However, implementing game-based learning tools and strategy requires careful thought to assure that instructors optimally align learning objectives with new technology. While we briefly discussed this earlier, it is worth emphasizing again. Without such efforts, at best the result is a series of learning technologies that receive only limited use by a handful of faculty who are comfortable with them and some of the students they teach. Outcomes can be substantially worse if an additive approach to technology accumulation fails to effectively integrate new tools for learning. This can lead to a graveyard of technology-based solutions gathering dust in a classroom or closet. Perhaps worst of all, without adequate integration and support, new tools can lead to a muddled curriculum that causes consternation for faculty as students attempt to reconcile their expectations for more traditional instruction with the reality of new tools to which they are unaccustomed.

The rising tide of digital resources has a powerful capacity to fundamentally transform and improve nursing and other forms of clinical education. However, early adopters who seek to stay on the cutting edge of clinical education would do well to ensure that they draw attention to both the power of digital media to advance clinical learning and the necessary and sufficient conditions that they must establish within a program to ensure that these new technologies are used effectively.

REFERENCES

Allan, S. (2010). The revolution of nursing pedagogy: A transformational process. *Teaching and Learning in Nursing, 5*(1), 33–38.

Bauman, E. (2007). *High fidelity simulation in healthcare.* PhD dissertation, The University of Wisconsin-Madison, United States. Dissertations & Theses @ CIC Institutions database. (Publication no. AAT 3294196 ISBN: 9780549383109 ProQuest document ID: 1453230861)

Bauman, E. (2010). Virtual reality and game-based clinical education. In K. B. Gaberson, & M. H. Oermann (Eds.), *Clinical teaching strategies in nursing education* (3rd ed.) New York: Springer Publishing Company.

Bauman, E. B., & Games, I. A. (2011). Contemporary theory for immersive worlds: Addressing engagement, culture, and diversity. In A. Cheney, & R. Sanders (Eds.), *Teaching and learning in 3D immersive worlds: Pedagogical models and constructivist approaches.* IGI Global.

Benner, P. (1984). *From novice to expert: Excellence and power in clinical nursing practice.* Menlo Park, CA: Addison-Wesley.

Benner, P., Tanner, C., & Chesla, C. (2009). *Expertise in nursing: Caring, clinical judgment, and ethics.* New York: Springer Publishing Company.

Bransford, J. D., & Schwartz, D. L. (1999). Rethinking transfer: A simple proposal with multiple implications. In A. Iran-Nejad, & P. D. Pearson (Eds.), *Review of research in education* (Vol. 24, pp. 61–101). Washington, DC: American Educational Research Association.

Brosterman, N. (1997). *Inventing kindergarten.* New York, NY: Harry N. Abrams, Inc.

Brown, J. S., Collins, A., & Duguid, P. (1989). Situated cognition and the culture of learning. *Educational Researcher, 18*(1), 32–42.

Brown, J. S., & Duguid, P. (2001). Knowledge and Organization: A social-practice perspective. *Organization Science, 12*(2), 198–213.

Brown, J. S. (2011). *Digital Media – New Learners of the 21st Century.* PBS, PBSVideo. Web. 28 Feb. 2011. http://video.pbs.org/video/1767466213/.

Browning, J. (1999). *Analysis of concepts and skills acquisition differences between web-delivered and classroom-delivered undergraduate instructional technology courses.* Dissertation Abstracts International, 60, 2456A. (ERIC Document Reproduction Service No. ADG 9938354).

Bryk, A. S., Rollow, S. G., & Pinnell, G. S. (1996). Urban School Development: Literacy as a lever for change. *Educational Policy, 10*(2), 172–201.

Bryk, A. S., Sebring, P. B., Kerbow, D., Rollow, S., & Easton, J. Q. (1998). Catalyzing basic organizational change at the building level. In A. S. Bryk, P. B. Sebring, D. Kerbow, S. Rollow, & J. Q. Easton (Eds.), *Charting Chicago school reform: Democratic localism as a lever for change* (pp. 93–129). Boulder, CO: Westview Press.

Campbell, S. H., & Daley, K. M. (2009). *Simulation scenarios for nurse educators: Making it real.* New York: Springer Publishing Company.

Cheney, A., & Sanders, R. L. (2011). *Teaching and learning in 3D immersive worlds: pedagogical models and constructivist approaches* (pp. 1–366). doi:10.4018/978-1-60960-517-9.

Collins, A., & Halverson, R. (2009). *Rethinking education in the age of technology: The digital revolution and the school.* New York, NY: Teachers College Press.

Cooper, J. B., & Taqueti, V. R. (2004). A brief history of the development of mannequin simulators for clinical education and training. *Quality and Safety in Health Care, 13*(Suppl. 1), i11–i18.

DeVita, M. (2005). Organizational factors affect human resuscitation: The role of simulation in resuscitation research. *Critical Care Medicine, 33*(5), 1150–1151.

Friedrich, M. J. (2002). Practice makes perfect: Risk-free medical training with patient simulators. *JAMA, 288*(22), 2808, 2811–2812.

Gaba, D. M. (2004). The future vision of simulation in health care. *Quality and Safety in Health Care, 13*(Suppl. 1), i2–i10.

Gaba, D. M., Howard, S. K., Fish, K., Smith, B., & Sowb, Y. (2001). Simulation-based training in anesthesia crisis resource management (ACRM): A decade of experience. *Simulation & Gaming, 32*(2), 175–193.

Games, I., & Bauman, E. (2011) Virtual worlds: An environment for cultural sensitivity education in the health sciences. *International Journal of Web Based Communities 7*(2), 187–205.

Gee, J. P. (2003). *What videogames have to teach us about learning and literacy.* New York, NY: Palgrave-McMillan.

Giddens, J. F., & Brady, D. F. (2007). Rescuing nursing education from content saturation: The case for a concept-based curriculum. *Journal of Nursing Education, 46*(2), 65–69.

Gordon, J. A., Oriol, N. E., & Cooper, J. B. (2004). Bringing good teaching cases "to life": A simulator-based medical education service. *Academic Medicine, 79*(1), 23–27.

Grenvik, A., & Schaefer, J. (2004). From resusci-anne to sim-man: The evolution of simulators in medicine. *Critical Care Medicine, 32*(Suppl. 2), S56–S57.

Halamek, L. P., Kaegi, D. M., Gaba, D. M., Sowb, Y. A., Smith, B. C., Smith, B. E. et al. (2000). Time for a new paradigm in pediatric medical education: Teaching neonatal resuscitation in a simulated delivery room environment. *Pediatrics, 106*(4), E45.

Halverson, R., Blakesley, C., & Figueiredo-Brown, R. (2011). Video game design as a model for professional learning. In M. S. Khine (Ed.), *Learning to play: Exploring the future of education with video games* (pp. 9–28). New York: Peter Lang.

Halverson, R., & Wolfenstein, M. (2007) Teacher evaluation game. Games for professional learning. Presented at UCEA 2007, November, 2007. Alexandria, VA.

Hammond, J., Bermann, M., Chen, B., & Kushins, L. (2002). Incorporation of a computerized human patient simulator in critical care training: A preliminary report. *Journal of Trauma Injury Infection and Critical Care, 53*(6), 1064–1067.

Helmreich, R. L. (2000). On error management: Lessons from aviation. *British Medical Journal, 320*(7237), 781–785.

Howard, S. K., Gaba, D. M., Smith, B. E., Weinger, M. B., Herndon, C., & Keshavacharya, S. et al. (2003). Simulation study of rested versus sleep-deprived anesthesiologists. *Anesthesiology, 98*(6), (6), 1345–1355, discussion 5A.

Kneebone, R. (2005). Evaluating clinical simulations for learning procedural skills: A theory-based approach. *Academic Medicine, 80*(6), 549–553.

Lane, J. L., Slavin, S., & Ziv, A. (2001). Simulation in medical education: A review. *Simulation & Gaming, 32*(3), 297–314.

Larew, C., Lessans, S., Spunt, D., Foster, D., & Covington, B. (2006). Innovations in clinical simulation: Application of benner's theory in an interactive patients care simulation. *Nursing Education Perspectives, 27*(1), 16–21.

Lave, J., & Wenger, E. (1991) *Situated learning: Legitimate peripheral participation.* New York, NY: Cambridge University Press.

Lee, S. K., Pardo, M., Gaba, D., Sowb, Y., Dicker, R., Straus, E. M. et al. (2003). Trauma assessment training with a patient simulator: A prospective, randomized study. *Journal of Trauma Injury Infection and Critical Care, 55*(4), 651–657.

Lofgren, E., & Fefferman, N. H. (2007). The untapped potential of virtual game worlds to shed light on real world epidemics. *The Lancet Infectious Diseases, 7,* 625–629.

Lynch, J., Aughwane, P., & Hammond, T. M. (2011). Video games and surgical ability: A literature review. *Journal of Surgical Education, 67*(3), 184–189.

McLellan, B. A. (1999). Early experience with simulated trauma resuscitation. *Canadian Journal of Surgery, 42*(3), 205–210.

Merriam, S. B., & Caffarella, R. S. (1999). *Learning in adulthood: A compressive guide* (2nd ed.) San Francisco: Jossey-Bass.

Merriam, S. B., & Caffarella, R. S. (2007). *Learning in adulthood: A compressive guide* (3rd ed.) San Francisco: Jossey-Bass.

Papert, S. (1980) *Constructionism vs. instructionism.* Speech delivered to an audience of educators in Japan.

Papert, S., & Harel, I. (1991). Situating constructionism. *Constructionism.* Norwood, NJ: Ablex.

Schaefer, J. J., III, & Grenvik, A. (2001). Simulation-based training at the university of Pittsburgh. *Annals of the Academy of Medicine, 30*(3), 274–280.

Shapiro, M. J., & Simmons, W. (2002). High fidelity medical simulation: A new paradigm in medical education. *Medicine & Health, Rhode Island, 85*(10), 316–317.

Sharpe, T., & Hawkins, A. (1998). Technology and the information age: A cautionary tale for higher education. *Quest, 50,* 19–32.

Shinnick, M. A., Woo, M. A., & Mentes, J. C. (2011). Human patient simulation: State of the science in prelicensure nursing education. *Journal of Nursing Education*, *50*(10), 65–72.

Shute, V. J. (2011). Stealth assessment in computer-based games to support learning. In S. Tobias, & J. D. Fletcher (Eds.), *Computer games and instruction*. Charlotte, NC: Information Age Publishers.

Squire, K. (2006). From content to context: Videogames as designed experience. *Educational Researcher*, *35*(8), 19–29.

Squire, K. (2011). *Video games & learning. Teaching and participatory culture in the digital age*. New York: Teachers College Press.

Squire, K. D., DeVane, B., & Durga, S. (2008). Designing centers of expertise for academic learning through video games. *Theory Into Practice*, *47*(3), 240–251.

Tan, G. M., Ti, L. K., Suresh, S., Ho, B. S., & Lee, T. L. (2002). Teaching first-year medical students physiology: Does the human patient simulator allow for more effective teaching? *Singapore Medical Journal*, *43*(5), 238–242.

Thomas, D., & Brown, J. S. (2011) *A new culture of learning: Cultivating the imagination for a world of constant change*. Self published. Printed by CreateSpace.

Tyczkowski, B., Bauman, E., Gallagher-Lepak, S., Vandenhouten, C., & Resop Reilly, J. (2012). An interface design evaluation of courses in a nursing program using an e-learning framework: A case study. In B. Khan (Ed.), *User interface design for virtual environments: Challenges and advances*. McWeadon Press: Washington, DC.

Vygotsky, L. (1978). *Mind in society*. Cambridge, MA: Harvard University Press.

Wolfenstein, M. (2010) *Leadership at play: How leadership in digital games can inform the future of instructional leadership*. Doctoral dissertation, University of Wisconsin–Madison, Madison, WI.

Ziv, A., Wolpe, P. R., Small, S. D., & Glick, S. (2003). Simulation-based medical education: An ethical imperative. *Academic Medicine*, *78*(8), 783–788.

2

Digital and Multimedia Literacy: Understanding the Language for Game-Based Learning

ERIC B. BAUMAN AND ALLAN BARCLAY

INTRODUCTION

*T*he rise in the use of simulation-based (SB) and now game-based (GB) learning in higher education is increasing. This includes nursing education and other clinical sciences disciplines such as pre-licensure and continuing education. Scholarly literature thoroughly documents research promoting simulation as an acceptable and effective pedagogy (Cant & Cooper, 2010). Game-based learning in virtual environments is seeing rapid and substantive integration in kindergarten through 12th grade education, particularly in the area of science, technology, engineering, and math (STEM). It is now becoming more prevalent in college and university education, including nursing, and other clinical disciplines (Gaba, 2004; Kato, 2010; Maxman, 2010; Miller, Chang, Wang, Beier, & Klisch, 2011). Accreditation bodies and curriculum committees understand that technology-based education encompassing simulation and game-based learning pedagogies continues to grow. They now recommend that simulation and game-based learning pedagogies become integral parts of health sciences education (Barnes, Kacmarek, Kageler, Morris, & Durbin, 2011; Decker, Utterback, Thomas, Mitchell, & Sportsman, 2011; DeMaria, Levine, & Bryson, 2010; Gaba, 2004; Weaver, 2011).

With increasing frequency educators now devote resources to ever larger and more sophisticated simulation centers that move beyond mannikin-based simulation. These simulation centers integrate virtual and augmented reality learning experiences stemming from the serious games movement and game-based learning in general. Accreditation bodies now make recommendations and set standards on how simulation should and can be integrated into curricula (Issenberg & Scalese, 2008).

Historically, simulation occurring on a personal computer was called screen-based simulation. As screen-based simulation begins to provide a game experience for learners and educators it has largely been re-termed as game-based learning or serious gaming. At the same time, curriculum committees have begun to anticipate, interpret, and integrate the recommendations of accrediting bodies' requirements into existing curricula. Decisions related to integration will have far-reaching, long-term impact on educators (Issenberg, McGaghie, Petrusa, Gordon, & Scalese, 2005).

The taxonomy of emerging educational technology remains informal at best. Taxonomy related to clinical education continues to emerge and is a robust topic for discussion among clinical sciences educators and researchers across several prominent organizations and conferences. These organizations include the International Nursing Association for Clinical Simulation and Learning (INACSL), the Society for Simulation in Healthcare (SSH), and Games For Health (G4H). They are challenged by a lack of uniformity in terminology that results in two conditions: similar terms that mean different things, and different terms that mean the same thing. Establishing a common and accepted taxonomy for game-based learning and simulation will lead to more efficient and effective access to relevant information about the pedagogy. Further, accepted taxonomy will also allow academic functions such as literature reviews to become more robust without relying on keyword searching alone. This, in turn, will empower educational designers, teaching faculty, program managers, and researchers by providing them with powerful mechanisms to evaluate game-based learning and simulation tools and techniques.

BACKGROUND

Experts who research the effectiveness of simulation and game-based learning have been hampered by a lack of a common language to describe not only the physical tools of the domain, but also the phenomenon of the simulation or game experience itself. What experts in the field are beginning to agree on is that the elements that make for a good game also make for good simulation (Bauman, 2007; Gee, 2003). Those who study the elements of good simulation find that defining and discussing good gaming is often confusing. Different academic fields often define simulation in a way that situates the term too discretely. Unfortunately, many of these fields have not looked beyond the confines of their own discipline when formulating their definitions.

The term "simulation" itself is not new. Ören (2011) found some 100 different definitions for the term "simulation" or the combined terms of "modeling and simulation." Interestingly, Ören found this inconsistency in the context of the general modeling and simulation literature, not within literature specific to nursing or other forms of clinical education. Some of the definitions for simulation include the term "game" or "gaming." However, other definitions explicitly exclude principles of gaming from those of simulation. In other words, some scholars see games as something entirely different than simulation. This same challenge now exists within the domain of game-based learning found across the clinical sciences. The authors refer to simulation by way of example, because the pedagogy of simulation and game-based learning are closely related.

Simulation that involves and strives for task mastery and even behavioral change is most effective when it engages facets of game design (Bauman, 2007; Zyda, 2005). Many serious games used in professional training include some facet of simulation within their narrative. Even low-fidelity simulation that focuses on task training encompasses facets of game design by incorporating common game-based variables such as consequence, scoring, and narrative. Nursing education has a long history of integrating low-fidelity simulation and standardized patient simulation into its curriculum. However, beyond agreeing that a simulator is used in a simulated experience, little progress has been made in the area of taxonomy as it relates to simulation-based and now game-based learning in healthcare. The term "mannikin" provides one example of the inconsistency in language use found throughout simulation and game-based learning. There are three accepted spellings of the word "mannikin" used throughout industry and the academic literature (Gaba, 2006).

The term "mannequin" from the French language traditionally refers to a life-size full or partial representation of a person, used for the fitting or displaying of clothes, a common tool of the tailor or seamstress. The term "manikin" is often defined as a person short or very small in stature, and is sometimes historically defined as synonymous with the terms "dwarf" or "pygmy." The spelling "mannikin" is most often defined as an anatomical model used for teaching anatomy or other medical procedures.

The same nomenclature-related challenges exist when trying to establish a consistent academic language for game-based learning. For example, the term Non-Player Character (NPC), which represents a key function of game programming and does not exist outside of the game or virtual environment, is often defined by a variety of terms or inconsistently. NPCs are in-world characters with whom the player/learners' avatars interact. The role of the NPC is to promote fidelity and advance the narrative of the game. It is possible that players' interactions with NPCs are so authentic that they do not know if NPCs are a function of programming or are actually being played by a real person. Similarly the term "bot" or sometimes "chat-bot" stems from early work in artificial intelligence. It is often used as a term to represent automated software agents that behave in an autonomous manner. Bots were often used as early versions of non-player characters in text-based virtual worlds to simulate conversations with players immersed in the virtual or game environment (Bauman, 2010; Bauman & Games, 2011; Games & Bauman, 2011).

In the same way, some use the term "Player Character" (PC) interchangeably with the term "Avatar." Players, or in the case of serious games or game-based learning, enter the virtual world as a player character. The player character is represented in world or on screen as an avatar. In this sense, both an NPC and a PC can be represented by the presence of an in-world avatar.

By examining existing taxonomy now and defining nomenclature for new technology and pedagogy as it occurs, we provide a more consistent path for technology integration and evaluation for existing and new curricula. With a consistent language to define simulation and game-based learning for nursing and other forms of clinical education, we can take an academic approach to understanding or establishing the efficacy of educational interventions that stem from this technology. The dilemma of definitions and taxonomy exists whether one engages qualitative, quantitative, or mixed methods educational research. A common and accepted taxonomy provides administrators with the needed tools to drive budgets, evaluate staff performance, and evaluate the educational outcomes of their curriculum. Common academic *resource discovery tools* such as literature databases and search engines (for example, CINAHL, PubMed, Google Scholar) are more efficient when teachers, researchers, and scholars can depend on a common language to create, automate, and leverage computer applications that consistently work with accepted taxonomy convention. Better taxonomy supports both research and application of research results in clinical and educational environments.

Educators commonly integrate technology into nursing and other health sciences curricula. Historically, using technology with curricula has mirrored technological advances in clinical practice. Nursing is uniquely positioned to make substantial contributions to the development of a taxonomy that supports the rapidly emerging pedagogical processes related to simulation and game-based learning in the health sciences. Nursing has historically used processes supported by taxonomy to provide standard mechanisms of practice. The nursing process uses the standard taxonomy of nursing diagnoses as a means for nursing education and nursing practice (Blegen & Tripp-Reimer, 1997)

While a history of embracing technology in nursing education exists, the language used to describe this technology and the theory supporting it remains fragmented and incomplete. Additionally, developing a common language embracing the technology associated with both simulation and game-based learning is complex, but crucial because it crosses a variety of disciplinary boundaries (for instance nursing, medicine, education, engineering, and computer science). This chapter will continue to focus on the importance of advocating for standard language to help teachers and researchers synthesize a taxonomy that helps them make sense of terminology supported in the simulation and game-based learning literature, not only in the nursing literature, but across multiple disciplines spanning healthcare and other professions.

Further, a taxonomy to support the internal validity of game-based learning and simulation will support and advance research, indexing, curriculum design, and assessment.

Without a common language it will become increasingly difficult to communicate with administrators, educational designers, instructional technologists, and providers of content (often vendors) in order to meet curriculum objectives and learner expectations.

TAXONOMIES, FOLKSONOMIES, AND OTHER METHODS OF CLASSIFYING INFORMATION

With the advent of social media and Web 2.0, the ability for people to classify and organize their own information in shared spaces has exploded. Web 2.0 in general refers to web-based applications that help users share the content that they generate. Users often use social media applications to interact with others in the Web 2.0 environment. Tools that exemplify Web 2.0 include, but are not limited to blogs, wikis, media sharing sites, and even more commonly known social networking and media sites such as Facebook and Twitter (Eysenbach, 2008; Skiba, 2009). The ease of use of new software, information, and media tools, coupled with the natural social inclination for people to talk to each other as a matter of problem-solving strategy has far outstripped efforts to create structured and agreed upon language in communities of practice. Using the existing language, while at the same time evaluating the efficacy and applicability of emerging taxonomy presents both challenges and opportunities. The rest of this chapter provides perspective and strategy for educators who are beginning to embrace pedagogy that leverages simulation and game-based learning.

CONTROLLED VOCABULARIES, TAXONOMIES, AND ONTOLOGIES

The terms *controlled vocabulary*, *taxonomy*, and *ontology* are often used interchangeably (and often imprecisely). This can make attempts to clarify the language of professions and the disciplines found within them challenging. For our purposes, we propose the following definitions.

Controlled Vocabulary

A *controlled vocabulary* is a set of terms used to describe a concept or domain with precision. When you encounter the words "see this" or "use this" as a cue or reference in a traditional library card catalogue, the words refer to a standardized term considered equivalent to the term you are using, a synonym.

The PubMed search engine automatically substitutes search terms in this manner. For example, the term "cancer" is mapped to "neoplasm." The advanced user options within PubMed allow users to choose terms to be selected independently or in combination with mapped terms to expand or narrow search criteria. Limits are also based on controlled vocabulary to promote consistency in otherwise ambiguous concepts found within a domain. By establishing a controlled vocabulary for simulation and game-based learning, communication could be greatly enhanced to better meet the needs of most students, educators, and scholars seeking to inform their practice or experience when integrating simulation and game-based learning throughout curricula. Controlled vocabularies allow search engines to consistently and efficiently direct users to accurate information. Applying a controlled vocabulary to computer programs promotes the use of consistent menus and other interface elements that direct users and simplify the search process. In other words, controlled vocabularies allow for precision and consistency in communication.

Taxonomy

A *taxonomy* is more structured than a controlled vocabulary. A taxonomy enumerates the relationships between the descriptive terms in a hierarchical fashion. The Linnaean classification system of biological classification is a prime example of taxonomy (Linnæus, 1735). Organisms are part of a structured hierarchy (for example, kingdom, phylum, genus, species, and so forth). A taxonomy is more useful than a controlled vocabulary because it provides structures to improve clarity in describing how things relate to each other in the context of a large set of data or information. Taxonomy moves beyond reconciliation or basic agreement on common terms and addresses the relationship of one term to another. Taxonomies are helpful in organizing information for search and retrieval, and provide overlap with programming details required to build databases.

Existing Taxonomies

The nursing profession has a rich history of classification and taxonomy related to both practice and education. Learning to become a nurse includes mastery of the language of nursing practice. Many students struggle with and bemoan our insistence that as students and novices they are forced to learn the nursing process that requires an understanding of unfamiliar and precise clinical language. The language drives the process of synthesizing nursing diagnoses. Nurses must use both structured and colloquial language daily as a matter of professional practice.

The process of learning the precise and structured language of nursing is necessary and important from a variety of perspectives. In terms of access to information, educators use taxonomies to organize learning and knowledge management or classification systems that support practice, education, and research. Automated or electronic management systems do not handle ambiguity or inconsistency well. People, to their credit, are much more adept at reconciling inconsistency and ambiguity. Examples of structured classification systems for nursing language include the following examples:

- CINAHL subject headings
- Nursing Problem List Subset of SNOMED CT
- International Classification for Nursing Practice, 2.0
- NANDA Nursing Diagnoses: Definitions and Classification
- Nursing Interventions Classification
- Nursing Outcomes Classification, 3rd edition
- Perioperative Nursing Data Set Source
- Clinical Care Classification System

Following are other more general healthcare classification systems:

- MeSH—Medical Subject Headings from the National Library of Medicine
- Unified Medical Language System (UMLS—a metathesaurus including several of the previous examples)
- International Classification of Disease
- Current Procedural Terminology

These classification systems address both broad and specific elements of patient procedures and clinical events (for instance disaster management, triage, and so on), but are inadequate to deal with game-based learning and technology-based simulations found throughout nursing and clinical education in general. The language of game-based learning originates in education and learning theory. The language of simulation and now game-based learning found throughout the health sciences does not really deal with the complexities that are associated with other disciplines like engineering, though it haphazardly addresses nursing and more general taxonomies. These non-healthcare taxonomies are not cleanly crosswalked to those found in healthcare. Different types of clinical educators and scholars using the same equipment and procedures in the same location may describe them inconsistently.

When educators and scholars pick and choose terminology from a variety of discipline-specific sources they often end up with a mish-mash of semi-structured language fraught with ambiguity and inconsistency. This can lead to confusion in scholarly publications and during face-to-face communication in both clinical and educational environments. The result is a true "Tower of Babble" which may affect teaching and learning, patient safety, and clinical outcomes.

Ontology

An *ontology* is even more descriptive than a taxonomy. Ontologies describe a body of knowledge or domain and provide a set of consistent descriptive terms in a hierarchy. Ontologies flesh out the details to provide a better understanding of the terminology and the concepts associated with a given domain. Ontologies provide structure to facilitate different uses of the same domain-specific information. Uses of domain-specific information include, but are not limited to analysis, data sharing, faceted search functions or browsing capabilities.

Concepts in multiple domains may be described differently based on their function. For example, the word "mannikin" may have different descriptions in educational, clinical, and administrative databases in addition to variant spellings. An ontology allows users to crosswalk terms between domains and to see the different descriptions for the same term. This is helpful when collaboration takes place across professional boundaries. Users see the full breadth of a concept's meaning across the disciplinary spectrum while database designers can increase the likelihood of high precision and recall in user searches.

The International Classification for Nursing Practice (ICNP) available via the National Centers for Biomedical Computing's BioPortal (http://bioportal.bioontology.org/ontology/ICNP) is an example of an existing nursing ontology. The ICNP describes specific concepts inherent to nursing practice like Complication, Diagnostic Phenomenon, Process, Social Support, and so on. The site provides a detailed list of the terms, a browser to visualize the interrelationships of terms, and other helpful tools. The ICNP not only assists students, clinicians, and scholars in their practice, but also provides guidance in the development of new derivative ontologies.

Depending on institutional needs, any or all the classification systems discussed in this chapter are useful and necessary to advance the use of simulation and game-based learning for clinical education and research. Consistency of terms can be addressed with a *controlled vocabulary*. The structure and relationships of the terms are addressed in a *taxonomy*. When stakeholders are encouraged to share information, *ontologies* help address large, complex domains.

Folksonomies
The term *folksonomy* ("folk classification") was coined by information architect Thomas Vander Waal to describe "the user-created bottom-up categorical structure development" of language (Morville, 2005, p. 136). Folksonomies let communities of practice define language structure from the bottom up (Owen, 2010). Folksonomies derive from grassroots organizational efforts by people who are well versed and invested in a specific topic. The best-known example of folksonomy is the use of *tagging* to describe content. The social bookmarking site del.icio.us provides an example of tagging. Users create their own descriptive keywords or use ones programmatically suggested by

other users. Over time, a user-generated thesaurus of sorts emerges. Unlike top-down hierarchical language tools, folksonomies reflect how real people talk and describe things "in the wild." They also adapt more quickly than Medical Subject Headings (MeSH) or other structured languages described earlier in this chapter that are updated annually at best.

In his book *Glut: Mastering Information Through the Ages*, author Alex Wright (2007) suggests that the user-generated classification of information is the way things have always been done until fairly recently. Wright feels that the highly structured organization of information is a historical artifact of the Industrial Age and the rise of the public library. Melvil Dewey, an American librarian and inventor of the Dewey Decimal System was an advocate for efficiency in efforts to describe all human knowledge now and into the future. His assembly line approach to information classification led to a divergence from an innate practice based on actual human communication toward a consistent but more arbitrary or artificial approach. The divergence between these objective and subjective approaches to classification creates obvious challenges when trying to design systems suited to emerging technology.

Simulation and game-based learning continues to be professionally situated, but also socially situated (Gee, 2003; Squire, 2006; Squire, Giovanetto, DeVane, & Durga, 2005). By this we mean the language used to discuss the integration of simulation and game-based learning in nursing, and more broadly across all professional practice disciplines is experiential in nature (Bauman, 2007; Bauman, 2010; Bauman & Games, 2011; Games & Bauman, 2011). The language emerges to describe constantly changing new phenomenon, not historical phenomenon.

Wells, in his essay *World Brain* (1938), describes what sounds very much like the World Wide Web (www) of today. Wells believed organizing and making accessible all human knowledge could lead to a new age of peace and understanding. Wells thought this would be accomplished by developing and maintaining a permanent and well-organized encyclopedia to document new and changing information. He believed this encyclopedia should be an open resource available to all members of society, just as Melvil Dewey believed. The challenge with today's World Wide Web and projects existing within the virtual spaces created within it is related to management. How do we organize and access the world's information if the content is poorly described and not available online—especially if it is seldom used and of little or no commercial or academic value?

CONVERGENCE AND POSSIBLE FUTURE DIRECTIONS

How do we as educators and scholars resolve the bottom-up and top-down approaches to language used in the context of academia? There is no easy answer, but we present several possibilities here.

Top-down approaches to language management already exist and are in use in academic and clinical environments. The integration of billing codes and controlled vocabularies into electronic medical records serves as an example of a top-down approach to language management. The question and challenge before academic stakeholders who currently use top-down language management systems like controlled vocabularies is how can bottom-up approaches be used to inform formal language management systems? Sites like del.icio.us were originally developed for personal bookmark and information management, but are now being used for research. We argue that people can use tools like del.icio.us to leverage the vast amounts of information found online related to simulation and game-based learning. The results of bottom-up data mining can be incorporated into existing formal systems like *taxonomies* and *ontologies*. In this way "native" use of terminology begins to inform accepted and formal practices of classification.

Engaging the study of current language use among various professions embracing games and simulation will facilitate normative structuring and weighting of terms for electronic search algorithms. The population interested in games and simulation in healthcare is not as large as the population of Facebook (let alone the entire Internet, as is the case with Google). Though multiprofessional, the games and simulation user population is relatively discrete, smaller, and thus easier to identify and work with. While the task of encouraging a large, heterogeneous group of stakeholders to think, write, and speak consistently about games and simulation is daunting, it is worth pursuing. Consistent dialogue, feedback, and input by stakeholders will encourage consensus related to the pedagogy of games and simulation in healthcare. Codifying a consistent language based on common use and scholarly consensus will support academic and practice facets of nursing.

INFORMATION TECHNOLOGY CONSIDERATIONS

One of the main drivers behind the quest for better-structured language in nursing education arises from the need to integrate technology related to practice and trends in education across the curriculum. This now includes games and simulation. The need for improvement in the language of nursing and clinical sciences instruction began with the integration of *information technology* (IT) as a tool for educators to create and deliver curriculum. The need for improvement in language became more acute as technology began to move beyond the traditional roles associated with IT and began to include facets of *instructional design* (ID), including the realm of created environments. There are many familiar examples of IT that already use structured language found throughout healthcare and academic practice. Some examples include, but are not limited to electronic medical records (EMR), student records, treatment plans, and search and retrieval of documents. Information technology tools require structure to work; there simply is no workable way to build an automated system to deal with ambiguous information.

SEARCH

The general public and educators alike often use Google as an IT triumph when describing a successful approach to organizing and finding information. Unfortunately, Google is not an applicable example for many scenarios discussed in this chapter. Google has amassed an enormous amount of resource information and information about user behavior. The Google PageRank algorithm does a very good job of basic web searching (Brin & Page, 1998). However, the Google search engine is proprietary. Institutions can license the Google search engine technology, but cannot let developers from their institution "get under the hood" to modify it. Further, academic institutions lack the type and amount of information needed to create a Google-style search engine based on the complexities of user behavior for relatively small closed search and retrieval systems. Many smaller databases using controlled language are not sophisticated enough to gather the kind of information needed to dramatically improve their search and retrieval capabilities and the services that they provide to the communities of practice that they target.

Improving the standard simulation and game-based language so that it presents structured and consistent information allows for better and more precise retrieval of information. It also improves the presentation and organization of information gleaned from user search results. Easily found and organized information is important because it informs curriculum design, implementation, and evaluation. For example, a long list of searchable items is very inefficient when trying to quickly process search results. However, a faceted or filtered approach helps to create structure in the search process. Refining a search request by platform or facets like "virtual reality" and "screen based" provides much more structure than either facet or filter alone, and certainly more structure than simply using the search term of "game" or "game-based." Efficient searching, and combined browsing (for example "drilling down" or navigating to resources) is possible with well-structured, consistently labeled information. Both Amazon.com and Wine.com serve as examples of a faceted approach to efficient searching. An example of a work in progress specific to simulation and game-based learning in healthcare can be found with the Games and Simulation for Healthcare Portal hosted by the Ebling Library at the University of Wisconsin–Madison (http://healthcaregames.wisc.edu/).

INDEXING AND METADATA

Well-structured information is crucial to database search functions. Structured information allows searches to take place using efficient and effective algorithms. The different language tools discussed earlier in this chapter (controlled vocabularies and other structured language systems) often overlap. When these language tools are integrated into metasearch systems like the National Library of Medicine's United Medical Language System, searching across different databases becomes manageable and productive. *Crosswalking* of terms can also occur in custom-built applications using synonym rings and "did you mean" spelling or phonetic suggestions. By crosswalking we mean associating similar search terms with each other to improve information retrieval when using search engines, searchable databases, and even searches taking place across various databases.

USER INTERFACE DESIGN

Many powerful software tools are crippled by a poorly designed interface. For the purposes of this chapter and text, the term "interface" means how and where the user interacts with the electronic medium, software, or tool. A clear, consistent and helpful interface is essential for tool usability (Raskin, 2000). While Raskin (2000) wrote about the difficulties and challenges associated with human-computer interaction over a decade ago, many of his observations still hold true today. Without a well-designed and intuitive interface, powerful search engines and databases end up frustrating users instead of facilitating the transfer of information (Tyczkowski, Bauman, Gallagher-Lepak,Vandenhouten, & Resop Reilly, 2012).

Interface designers should not have to worry about language consistency, particularly across domains with a plethora of complex content. However, without a robust classification system, complex content can muddle the interface design process. Worse yet, if developers and designers do not effectively address content classification before and during the design process, end users will find the interface of search engines and other related electronic tools of little or no use.

Commercial website architects devote extensive resources to the development of consistent language to make a site more useful and usable to their audience. Because systems of classification already exist across academia, it should be possible to adapt existing tools and their related interface systems for game-based learning more efficiently and effectively than creating entirely new systems from scratch. Existing tools support integrative automation of new information. This approach is more effective, efficient, and less expensive than creating new databases from scratch.

Examples of helpful interface design include drop-down pick lists or auto-complete functions found in search boxes or other navigational elements of databases. These relatively simple additions to the interface speed up task completion, while systematically refining searches. Use of consistent language is both encouraged and refined though good interface design. Additional supplemental context-sensitive pearls, tips, and scope notes should be made available as part of the interface tool to assure users are engaging terms consistently and in ways that represent conventional and expected meaning.

HARDWARE AND SOFTWARE PURCHASING AND MANAGEMENT

There are many things to consider when making decisions related to the purchase of simulation and game-based technology. Consideration should include hardware and software requirements such as platform, processor specifications, manufacturer, memory, and cost. High-fidelity mannikins will involve both hardware and software. The hardware and software for mannikin-based simulators is generally proprietary and not easily substituted in terms of features or functions. However, game-based technology often, but not always, exists as a function of software that may or may not be compatible with certain operating platforms (for example, Mac, PC or Unix) or hardware (such as graphics processing unit, processor speed, or memory). Users of simulation and game-based technology should acknowledge that hardware and software are often brand or platform specific and not necessarily interoperable or interchangeable.

Purchasing the right hardware and software should begin with a well thought out discussion and analysis of curriculum objectives. When you consider this analysis along with administrative and cost considerations you quickly accumulate a large and complicated amount of information. Computer hardware has standardized language to describe its attributes, as does software. However, if language describing educational criteria and objectives are inconsistent, making informed decisions about educational relevance and fit related to hardware and software is very challenging. In other words, the hardware and software (whether mannikin-based or game-based) are tools to deliver the educational experience, not drive it. Consistent use of language will assist stakeholders the process of acquiring technology that supports curriculum objectives.

Once learning spaces have been built to facilitate simulation and game-based learning experiences, whether these spaces exist in physical or virtual environments, they need to be maintained and updated. This often requires both hardware and software updating. Further, all use of these spaces and the learning experiences that take place in them should be tracked for evaluation or assessment. When standardized language is used to describe the hardware, software, and learning experiences taking place in created spaces, it is possible to maintain a curriculum rich in emerging technology, while systematically evaluating the effectiveness of any given educational intervention.

Boundary crossing and multiprofessional education should be considered when purchasing and managing equipment. Simulation and game-based learning provide unique opportunities to provide authentically situated experiences that mirror actual practice (Bauman, 2010; Bauman & Games, 2011; Gaba, 2004; Games & Bauman, 2011). If one accepts this premise, it becomes clear that an investment in simulation and game-based learning is by its very nature multidisciplinary. Educators from different but related fields in healthcare must find common language to express desired learning processes and outcomes. Administrators and business managers need to be able to make decisions based on financial and logistical criteria while meeting the needs of nursing and other allied health educators. Further, administrators from different departments and schools often use central procurement plans that do not have a full or robust knowledge of individual departmental needs. The multistep process inherent to purchasing in academic and clinical institutions that sits between the educator and the product can be a very challenging task to deal with. A structured language specific to simulation and game-based learning for clinical education will facilitate communication and understanding among representative stakeholders including educators, administrators, and vendors. This will in turn simplify the product procurement process.

Language and taxonomy discrepancies also exist among vendors who are supplying products for the simulation and game-based learning market. This exists in part because specific products providing similar experiences have intellectual property protections. Companies go to great lengths to brand their products as different from others in the marketplace. Often educators must make decisions about purchasing products based on vendor-supplied materials that are not consistent across the industry. Marketers describe most products using ambiguous marketing language or based on a discrete function rather than educational experiences that the product tries to support. A standardized vocabulary ought to address basic product function, a target audience, or discipline, and actual learning outcomes drawn directly from stakeholders' curriculums. A standard vocabulary assures a good fit for technology integration affecting high stakes elements of curriculum and program accreditation. Language standardization also provides an interesting feedback loop so that customers, educators, and vendors can effectively study and rate how technology objectively meets learner objectives.

THEORETICAL CASE STUDY: THE NEW ACADEMIC CLINICAL SIMULATION LAB

The University Foundation has made a generous donation for the creation of a new simulation lab at the mythical Miskatonic University School of Nursing. The school is eager to impress donors and peers at other institutions. The School of Nursing is putting a great deal of effort into making sure all aspects of educational games and simulation are available to students in the new laboratory. The school plans to include high-fidelity mannikin simulators, task trainers, computer-based training, and *serious games*. The Foundation's gift represents a one-time capital gift and subsequent gifts are unlikely. The school plans to purchase the best equipment and make sure that it is well integrated into their curriculum. They are developing a plan to manage and maintain the physical space and all of their new equipment. Further, the school plans to develop a robust research program that yields significant recognition through scholarly publication. In other words, the School of Nursing wants to make sure that the University Foundation, its donors, and the campus administrators are pleased with how the Foundation's money is spent. Below we provide discussion illustrating the importance and implications of how language and taxonomy can be leveraged to enhance process.

INITIAL EQUIPMENT, SOFTWARE, AND BEST PRACTICES RESEARCH

The following questions frame and inform a useful process for the acquisition of simulation and game-based technology. What equipment and software is available and what will it cost? What software or hardware requirements exist? Will other schools or departments share equipment ownership outside of the School of Nursing? If so, how will this be supported? Are there any preexisting relationships among vendors? Are there plans to develop software in-house, and if so will it be shared in any way and who will own it?

Taxonomy and Language Implications

The language that companies use to describe game-based technology, simulators, and software should assist stakeholders with purchasing decisions. Different companies often use different terminology to describe their brand. Trademarked language is sometimes used to define both very similar and very different products. For example, CAE Healthcare (formally known as Medical Technologies Incorporated or METI) uses the word or term Müse® to define their operating system. Müse® software is proprietary and can only be used to drive CAE Healthcare/METI simulators. Similarly, the SimMan® mannikin-based simulator is a proprietary simulator developed by Laerdal Medical Corporation. While these products share some similarities, they are not interchangeable and are in fact two very different products. The *NOELLE®* mannikin-based simulator is very different from the Laerdal SimMan®. The *NOELLE®* simulator is a birthing simulator and neither the *NOELLE®* nor the SimMan® is compatible with the Müse® software. This example demonstrates the need to understand the importance of language in the context of simulation and game-based learning and further exemplifies why nursing and other clinical instructors embracing this type of technology should move toward a standard taxonomy or controlled language.

CURRICULUM AND CLINICAL INTEGRATION

Faculty stakeholder identification is one of the most important aspects related to designing, building, and integrating simulation and game-based learning into a curriculum. In our hypothetical case study, faculty should identify existing courses that are best suited to leverage the school's new resources. Faculty should also start to make decisions about how game and simulation-based technology should inform new courses and engage students in meaningful ways.

Other areas to address in the context of this case study include identifying how new technology can meet specific skill and experience needs of students. In other words, how can the school use the new lab to identify and address gaps in the existing curricula that will promote student success and program accreditation?

Identifying current instructors who have experience with educational games or simulation will provide new programs with built-in champions who are familiar with game and simulation pedagogy. Faculty should consider evaluation processes to document student experiences and achievements that take place in the lab using the new technology as a mechanism for future research. Novel opportunities like virtual practice e-portfolios provide a way for students and faculty to demonstrate situated student proficiency. As the reader can see, there are a myriad of questions and facets related to curriculum design, implementation, integration, and evaluation that should be addressed when integrating simulation and game-based learning into nursing and other clinical curricula.

Taxonomy and Language Implications

Consistent use of language throughout any curriculum or across related curricula allows for stakeholders to track the following:

- Educational experiences
- Continuing educational experiences
- Variations between instructors, schools, or institutions

For example, if local hospitals are using a specific term to define a learning objective while the nursing school uses a different term to define the same objective, a database using controlled language or a relevant taxonomy can reconcile these differences before educational experiences occur. Reconciling language discrepancies that map to educational objectives and entry to practice supports students during their transition from student to clinician.

It is challenging to meet curriculum objectives and accrediting standards while meeting the needs of community stakeholders. Stakeholders, including potential employers for new graduates often have institutional standards of practice that may vary those found in academic nursing curricula. A standard language for simulation and game-based learning has the potential to provide consistency and understanding for learners as they make the very important and challenging transition from novice to expert (Bauman, 2007; Bauman, 2010; Benner, 1984; Benner, Tanner, & Chesla, 2009).

LAB USAGE AND RESOURCE MANAGEMENT

The relatively large capital and ongoing expense of technology-facilitated learning requires robust and ongoing resource management analysis. This analysis includes aspects of scheduling and access for both physical and virtual environments. This analysis should include all stakeholders, including those residing outside of the School of Nursing:

- Will the local School of Medicine or local hospitals be interested in leveraging the resources available through the new lab?
- Will other departments (education and sciences) and members of the public (K12 education, fire departments, and first responders) have an interest in the lab and should they be considered stakeholders?
- Will equipment circulate outside the lab like laptops or tablet computers, game consoles, or simulators themselves?
- Will any software be distributed for use on student- or instructor-owned equipment?

If so, then stakeholders should consider cost sharing and instructional technology support for shared resources.

Taxonomy and Language Implications

Stakeholders using the same language will be better positioned to discuss collaborative opportunities, including inter-professional learning and research. Common language usage allows instructional designers and technologists to meet and support expectations of internal and external stakeholders efficiently and effectively.

PROMOTION, PUBLICATIONS, AND RESEARCH

How people use language will have a profound effect on promotion of the new lab. Descriptions of undergraduate and graduate level courses in the timetable and syllabi will drive interest, stakeholder perceptions, and the ability to leverage technology to its maximum potential. The way educators describe courses for professional learners will drive the lab's continuing education program and budget. Immediate promotion of the lab will depend on creating, documenting, and exemplifying user satisfaction. In the early operational stages of any new lab, word of mouth will be one of the most cost effective and immediate avenues for promotion. As the lab moves beyond the singular scope of education and begins to support research, the language used to describe what is taking place in conjunction with the lab and its technology becomes even more important, even essential.

Taxonomy and Language Implications

Using a structured language helps administrators and educators define course objectives and ensure a curriculum is clear and consistent. It also informs research and publication goals. Structured language allows you to evaluate existing resources and provides direction for storing and archiving emerging teaching and research artifacts. At stake is not merely your lab's own research, but the ability to interpret and repeat others' research. New requirements from funding agencies for research data preservation, management, and sharing will also be relevant to lab management practices. In order to interpret, repeat, and later describe your technique and the techniques of others working in the discipline of simulation and game-based learning in nursing and more broadly, healthcare, you must move toward standards that are defined consistently by accepted taxonomy (Schaefer et al., 2011).

In a very discrete example, a large midwestern university developed a simulation-based resuscitation and crisis management course for students in their senior year. The course incorporated components of the American Heart Association (AHA) Advanced Cardiac Life Support (ACLS) curriculum. The AHA ACLS curriculum is an essential component of many hospitals' credentialing process. This course became popular with students. However, the stand-alone AHA ACLS curriculum is traditionally seen as a continuing education course for licensed and experienced clinicians. Unfortunately, teaching faculty and staff often referred to this immersive and very comprehensive simulation and multimedia-based course as simply ACLS, instead of its full syllabus name, "Resuscitation and Crisis Management." This caused much confusion among students and administrators as to what the actual course content was, and what it should be.

EVALUATION AND ASSESSMENT

Whether a new lab or learning environment focuses primarily on teaching or aspires to develop a robust research program, evaluation and assessment is important to the success of your lab. Faculty and other instructors are generally comfortable assessing student performance. However, assessing performance in a new mixed or multimedia environment often represents a paradigm shift for many teachers. Errors or wrong answers become opportunities for improvement; they are the experiential part of learning. How learners are assessed in circumstances where we expect failure, recovery, and performance remediation often requires teachers to look beyond the traditional nursing curricula to explain performance-based behavioral change.

Taxonomy and Language Implications

When leveraging mixed and multimedia technology in educational contexts, it is important to continually evaluate the teaching medium (simulation and game-based learning) and the objective to technology fit. It is also important to evaluate individual teachers' success as facilitators in the mixed and multimedia environment. Later chapters of this book will provide a more in-depth discussion of evaluation and assessment. The point emphasized here is that language and taxonomy are able to provide a high level of sophistication and consistency in your assessment and evaluation processes (Schaefer, et al., 2011).

EXERCISE

Using the Miskatonic case study discussion above, try to imagine yourself in their situation. Ask yourself the following questions:

• How would you respond to the task of developing a new simulation lab? Are there elements in your setting not addressed here? You could also explore this case study as a "forensic" exercise for existing labs.
• Are you aware of any recently developed labs, perhaps even at your institution? If so, how are they addressing the issues discussed in the case study? Can you identify any problems that could have been addressed by use of well-structured language?
• Can you identify any lab functions that took advantage of structured language, and did it streamline or inform educational or operational processes effectively?

SUMMARY

In this chapter we have expressed the importance of consistent language and how it supports educational scholarship, particularly when scholarship engages emerging technology such as simulation and game-based learning. We have stressed that simulation and game-based learning, while often used as an emerging educational modality, is by definition most effective when pursued from a multidisciplinary or multiprofessional perspective. It is mutually inclusive of other disciplines including, but not limited to, educational technology, engineering, computer and information sciences, and adult education. From this perspective, reinventing the language for each discipline is not only time consuming and frustrating, but also we argue that reinventing the language of simulation and game-based learning actually hampers academic scholarship.

We have discussed several approaches related to language consistency and validity as approaches for clarifying the language of simulation and game-based learning for nursing and other clinical education disciplines found in healthcare. We defined and discussed how stakeholders can use taxonomies, ontologies, controlled vocabularies, and folksonomies to reconcile inconsistent but similar terms within and across disciplines.

We also provided a discussion of why language matters from various management perspectives associated with simulation and game-based learning. In an attempt to situate the discussion, we provided a theoretical case study about the development of a proposed new simulation laboratory. In this case study we provided the reader with concrete examples of where structured and consistent language could be leveraged to optimize the promotion, productivity, and assessment of a lab itself, as well as the products of the lab, whether those products are focused on education, research, or some combination of the two.

REFERENCES

Barnes, T. A., Kacmarek, R. M., Kageler, W. V., Morris, M. J., & Durbin, C. G. (2011). Transitioning the respiratory therapy workforce for 2015 and beyond. *Respiratory Care, 56*(5), 681–690.

Bauman, E. (2007). *High fidelity simulation in healthcare.* PhD dissertation, The University of Wisconsin-Madison, United States. Dissertations & Thesis @ CIC Institutions database (Publication no. AAT 3294196).

Bauman, E. (2010). Virtual reality and game-based clinical education. In K. B. Gaberson, & M. H. Oermann (Eds.), *Clinical teaching strategies in nursing education* (3rd ed). New York: Springer Publishing Company.

Bauman, E. B., & Games, I. A. (2011). Contemporary theory for immersive worlds: Addressing engagement, culture, and diversity. In A. Cheney, & R. Sanders (Eds.), *Teaching and learning in 3D immersive worlds: Pedagogical models and constructivist approaches.* Hershey, Pa: IGI Global.

Benner, P. (1984). *From novice to expert: Excellence and power in clinical nursing practice.* Menlo Park, CA: Addison-Wesley.

Benner, P., Tanner, C., & Chesla, C. (2009). *Expertise in nursing: Caring, clinical judgment, and ethics.* New York: Springer Publishing Company.

Blegen, M. A., & Tripp-Reimer, T. (1997). Implications of nursing taxonomies for middle-range theory development. *Advances in Nursing Science, 19*(3), 37–49.

Brin, S., & Page, L. (1998). The anatomy of a large-scale hypertextual web search engine. In Seventh International World-Wide Web Conference (WWW1998), April 14–18, 1998. Brisbane, Australia.

Cant, R. P., & Cooper, S. J. (2010). Simulation-based learning in nurse education: Systematic review. *Journal of Advanced Nursing 66*(1), 3-15.

Decker, S., Utterback, V. A., Thomas, M. B., Mitchell, M., & Sportsman, S. (2011). Assessing continued competency through simulation: A call for stringent action. *Nursing Education Perspectives, 32*(2), 120-125.

Demaria, S., Levine, A. I., & Bryson, E. O. (2010). The use of multi-modality simulation in retraining of the physician for medical lisensure. *Journal of Clinical Anesthesia, 22*(4), 294-299.

Eysenbach, G. (2008). Medicine 2.0: Social networking, collaboration, participation, apomediation, and openness. *Journal of Medical Internet Research, 10*(3), e22.

Gaba, D. M. (2004). The future vision of simulation in health care. *Quality and Safety in Health Care, 13*(Suppl. 1), i2-i10.

Gaba, D. M. (2006). What's in name? A mannequin by any other name would work as well. *Simulation in Healthcare, 1*(2), 64-65.

Games, I., & Bauman, E. (2011). Virtual worlds: An environment for cultural sensitivity education in the health sciences. *International Journal of Web Based Communities, 7*(2), 189-205.

Gee, J. P. (2003). *What video games have to teach us about learning literacy.* New York: Palgrave MacMillian.

Issenberg, S., McGaghie, W. C., Petrusa, E. R., Gordon, D., & Scalese, R. J. (2005). Features and uses of high-fidelity medical simulations that lead to effective learning: A BEME systematic review. *Medical Teacher, 27*(1), 10-28.

Issenberg, S. B., & Scalese, R. J. (2008). Simulation in health care education. *Perspectives in Biology and Medicine, 51*(1), 31-46.

Kato, P. M. (2010). Video games in health care: Closing the gap. *Review of General Psychology, 14*(2), 113-121.

Linnæus, C. (1735). Systema naturæ, sive regna tria naturæ systematice proposita per classes, ordines, genera, & species. Lugduni Batavorum.

Maxman, A. (2010). Video games and the second life of science class. *Cell, 141*(2), 201-203.

Miller, L. M., Chang, C. I., Wang, S., Beier, M. E., & Klisch, Y. (2011). Learning and motivational impacts of a multimedia science game. *Computers & Education, 57*, 1425-1433.

Morville, P. (2005). *Ambient findability: What we find changes who we become.* [1st ed.]. Sebastopol, CA: O'Reilly Media.

Ören, T. (2011). The any acets of simulation through a collection of about 100 definitions. *SCS M&S Magazine, 2011*(2), 82-92.

Owen, K. (2010). Critical success factors in the development of folksonomy-based knowledge management tools. *In* T. Dumova, & R. Fiordo (Eds.), *Handbook of research on social interaction technologies and collaboration: Concepts and trends.* Hershey, PA: IGI Global.

Raskin, J. (2000). *The humane interface: New directions for designing interactive systems.* Indianapolis, IN: Addison-Wesley Professional.

Schaefer, J., III, Vanderbilt, A., Cason, C., Bauman, E., Glavin, R., Lee, F. et al. (2011). Literature review: Instructional design and pedagogy science in healthcare simulation. *Simulation in Healthcare, 6*(7), S30-S41, doi: 10.1097/SIH.0b013e31822237b4

Skiba, D. J. (2009). Nursing Practice 2.0: The wisdom of crowds. *Nursing Education Persectives, 30*(3), 191.

Squire, K. (2006). From content to context: Videogames as designed experience. *Educational Researcher, 35*(8), 19–29.

Squire, K., Giovanetto, L., DeVane, B., & Durga, S. (2005). From users to designers: Building a self-organizing game-based learning environment. *Technology Trends, 49*(5), 34–42.

Tyczkowski, B., Bauman, E., Gallagher-Lepak, S., Vandenhouten, C., & Resop Reilly, J. (2012). An interface design evaluation of courses in a nursing program using an e-learning framework: A case study. In B. Khan (Ed.), *User interface design for virtual environments: Challenges and advances*. Washington, DC: McWeadon Press.

Weaver, A. (2011). High-fidelity patient simulation in nursing education: An integrative review. *Nursing Education Perspectives, 32*(1), 37–40.

Wells, H. G. (1938). *World brain*. Garden City, NY, Doubleday: Doran and Co, Inc.

Wright, A. (2007). *Glut: mastering information through the ages*. Washington, DC: Joseph Henry Press.

Zyda, M. (2005). From visual simulation to virtual reality games. *Computer, 38*(9), 25–32.

3

Virtual Learning Spaces: Using New and Emerging Game-Based Learning Theories for Nursing Clinical Skills Development

BEN DEVANE AND ERIC B. BAUMAN

OVERVIEW

*S*hunned in educational circles a decade ago, digital games and simulations have recently been embraced as effective learning tools in mainstream educational, scientific, corporate, and policy-making circles. Institutions and companies as diverse as the National Academy of Sciences, McGraw-Hill, the U.S. Department of Education, and Kaiser Permanente now look to games and simulations as a powerful educational medium. Games and simulations, scholarship finds, have the potential to help educators build meaningful and compelling learning experiences that guide learners into deeper and more nuanced understandings of learning domains.

However, powerful institutions and organizations have embraced games and simulations in a manner that is at odds with the way in which they truly help people learn. Research often frames game- and simulation-based learning environments as "teaching machines" that efficiently transmit information to passive learners, rather than as sociocognitive tools that helps enhance the quality of experiential learning in rich educational contexts. Worse still, emerging behaviorist paradigms treat games and simulations purely as a means of behavior change, akin to cheese in a maze for a mouse. Unfortunately, when games and simulations are used in nursing and health sciences education, they are often designed, implemented, and understood as teaching machines or instruments of behavior change that replace and supersede existing curriculum and instruction, instead of enhancing and transforming it.

In this chapter, we argue that good learning games and simulations, however, are not "teaching machines," as B.F. Skinner (1957) termed them, that efficiently pump information into the mind of the learner. Rather, they are "designed experiences" (Squire, 2006). Designed experiences existing in created environments (Games & Bauman, 2011) are digital participation structures that help a person learn by *experiencing knowledge* through action in a *context-rich* environment.

This chapter describes how the designed experiences framework for learning games and simulations grows out of an *experiential learning* perspective, that holds that people learn best through doing (C.F. Dewey, 1916). Accordingly, in designed experiences "participants learn through a grammar of *doing* and *being*" (Squire, 2006, p. 24). These well-crafted experiences guide learners through new knowledge domains, introduce them to new context-dependent skills in a meaningful domain situated context, and present them with problem-solving opportunities with consequential feedback that allow learners to test the limits of their new capabilities.

There are very different visions about what learning games and simulations should do, because there are very different and sometimes competing existing theories about how people think and learn. Different theories treat information-processing from behaviorist and experiential perspectives. In this chapter we argue that we should design games and simulations as "designed experiences" but not rooted in an "information processing" theory of mind where learning is seen as a matter of information streaming into the brain. Further, "designed experiences" are not descended from a "behaviorist" theory of mind that sees human learning as a matter of punishing bad actions and rewarding good ones, as famed behavioral psychologist B.F. Skinner did with laboratory animal experiments (see Skinner, 1957). Instead, the "designed experiences" framework grows out of the century-old theory of "experiential learning," that understands learning to consist of context-specific and socially situated cycles of meaningful action and reflection (Squire, 2006; Squire, DeVane, B., & Durga, 2008). Coincidentally or not, nursing education and game-based learning paradigms share this experiential learning foundation. Both have historically emphasized learning through experience, practice and mentorship in authentic or convincing contexts.

Designed experiences, and experiential learning more generally, bear a curious resemblance to major paradigms in nursing education. Designed experiences relate to nursing education through the trajectory of experiential learning theory, the foundation of the designed experiences framework, from its inception in the work of John Dewey, and follow it through to examine the influence of the reflective practice in nursing and education through meaningful action in learning games. Digital games and simulations are powerful learning tools because they provide learners with opportunities to experience trying out new knowledge and skills in a "safe" space, and a structure for reflecting on those experiences that makes them meaningful and memorable. Experiential learning in these spaces is a result of action and reflection in a consequential and purpose-driven context. Such a framework for learning is very different from behaviorist and information processing models of the mind and learning.

This chapter first explains the relevance of designed experiences to clinical education. It then outlines the roots of the "designed experiences" framework in experiential learning theory, and then traces the history of the relationship between experiential learning, reflective practice and clinical nursing education. Finally, this chapter describes in detail the features of game-based designed experiences that are relevant to education, and argues that these mechanics resolve historical pedagogical problems in educational paradigms, like the "reflective practice" (Schön, 1983) and "thinking in action" (Benner, 1984) of nursing that grow out of experiential learning theory. This chapter argues that influential paradigms in nurse education and learning games actually bear a curious resemblance, and that the two fields confront many of the same problems in teaching and learning.

LEARNING GAMES AND SIMULATIONS IN CLINICAL ENVIRONMENTS

For professionals who work in clinical environments, games and simulations hold great promise as a learning and practice tool. They offer a model of learning and reflection that are unique among digital learning tools, many of which are built on a "transmission model" of learning (DeVane & Squire, 2008). Games and simulations are different in that they have two features that Powerpoint slides, interactive quizzes, and other electronic instructional methods do not: they are *experiential* and *context-rich* (Games & Bauman, 2011; Squire, 2006). These two features of games and simulations make them more similar to older models of teaching and learning—like clinical supervision and professional mentorship—than they are to digital methods of teaching used by instructional designers. Experiential and context rich features of games and simulations offer the possibility of learning through the simulation of meaningful action—they offer the ability to experiment with action and solutions in a "safe" space where the consequences of failure are lessened but success is rewarded. Bauman (2010) articulates the implications these features of games and simulations have for nurse education:

> The designed clinical learning activity can provide nursing students with important professional cues related to the conduct associated with the profession that they are seeking to join. In addition, the focus on learning through designed learning activities allows teachers to guide students within situated contexts of practice that are relevant to specific clinical areas
>
> —*Games & Bauman, 2011; Gee, 2003*

The context-rich nature of games and simulations can provide detailed but not wholly authentic models of the situations that nursing students and apprentices will encounter in clinical settings. These situational models provide players with practice spaces in which to try out acquired skills and dis-cover new ones in a controlled environment that does not overwhelm them with the messy details of authentic nursing. It is not that we are trying to protect students from actual clinical practice, rather we hope to provide them contextually relevant practice spaces in ways that manage the confound-ing variables often present when immersing an uninitiated student into an existing day-to-day practice.

Learning games and simulations provide players with virtual "practice fields" that provide them with opportunities for problem-solving and skill execution in a controlled setting as well as a sense of safety in that there are lessened social consequences (Barab & Duffy, 2000; Gee, 2007; Games & Bauman, 2011; DeVane Durga, & Squire, 2010). Bauman (2010) describes how the psychosocial moratorium that games provide has implications for nursing:

> In general, traditional simulation-based education has been helpful in preparing students for technical skill development and advanced clinical learning, and in preparation for independent practice. Simulation is most often employed throughout the health professions, including nursing, to prepare students for situations that involve high risk but occur infrequently (DeVita, 2005; Gaba, Howard, Fish, Smith, & Sowb, 2001; Helmreich, 2000). Management of complex, high-risk patient care situations such as trauma resuscitation, cardiac resuscitation, and crisis management have traditionally been taught through didactic preparation, followed by direct hands-on learning activities (Gaba, 2004; Lee et al., 2003; McLellan, 1999). Real-life learning activities cannot be produced on demand, nor is it ethical or feasible to allow students to direct the care of patients in crisis (Flanagan, Nestel, D., & Josep, 2004; Friedrich, 2002; Hammond, 2004). This raises the important question of how to adequately teach and prepare for crises that we know will occur during clinical learning activities and future professional practice.
> —*Bauman, 2010, pp. 187–188*

It is difficult, in other words, to physically reproduce the real-world experiences, activities, and contexts that nursing students need to prepare for in the actual clinical environment. Moreover, it is not ethical or desirable for student or patient outcome to introduce students to actual practice *in situ*, par-ticularly in emergencies and other low-incidence, high-risk clinical encounters. This predicament leads to nursing students being taught about the most dire and important challenges they will face in clinical practice through direct verbal instruction rather than through context-rich experiences.

Studies of expertise and organization have estimated that it takes 10,000 hours of real world practice for a person to develop from novice to expert in any given domain activity (Ericsson et al., 1993; Gladwell, 2008). Expertise in a given field requires many hours of knowledgeable and deliberate practical experience (for example triaging and treating severely injured patients) in a set of similar contexts (such as hospital emergency rooms). Benner (1984) posited that it took some 7 years for the novice nurse to progress to a state of expertise. While nurses entering into clinical practice are not expected to be experts, one might expect that nursing students would have a substantive amount of clinical experience. Instead, nursing students are presented with hours of verbal instruction about what they should do in often-critical situations. Didactic verbal instruction about the critically important activities of nursing practice does a disservice to nursing students, leaving them with little real-world experience on which to draw. Bauman (2010) articulates the problem thusly:

> Unfortunately, students are not exposed to all of the relevant clinical educational opportunities needed to prepare them for the transition from novice to expert (Benner, 1984; Larew, Lessans, Spunt, Foster, & Covington, 2006). This is not to imply that graduate nurses should enter the profession as experts, but rather, new graduates or novice clinicians ought to be poised to enter nursing as a profession with valuable experiences on which to build as they strive for clinical expertise. Clinical encounters of educational value need not be left to chance; rather, these situations can be created and designed through simulation-based technology, including *virtual reality* and *web-based environments*, to ensure that all students have the opportunity to achieve desired learning outcomes (Bauman, 2007; Campbell & Daley, 2009; Friedrich, 2002; Games & Bauman, 2011; Gordon, Oriol, & Cooper, 2004; Lane, Slavin, & Ziv, 2001; Shapiro & Simmons, 2002; Ziv, Wolpe, Small, & Glick, 2003).
> —*Bauman, 2010, p. 184*

The context-rich, *designed experiences* of learning games and simulation provide robust tools for nursing students to begin developing expertise through simulated real-world practice. They are structured spaces that simulate authentic practice, so that learners can begin to develop expertise in constrained but meaningful contexts for activity.

Critics complain that the theory of designed experiences lacks detail and definition. Moreover, they argue, the designed experiences framework seems ungrounded in any specific intellectual or research tradition. This chapter aims to address those criticisms by describing in detail both learning with designed experiences and its intellectual genealogy. The latter exercise is particularly important when we think about the relationship between designed experiences and nursing education. In fact, designed experiences share a scholarly history with "reflective practice" framework for nursing pedagogy (Benner 1984; Schön, 1983).

Though learning games and simulations are relatively recent phenomena, the theory of designed experiences, as well as reflective practice, come out of a century-old tradition of experiential learning pedagogy, brought to prominence by the late philosopher and educator John Dewey (see Dewey, 1902, 1926, 1938). In addition, influential educational paradigms in nursing also grow out of this well-known pedagogical paradigm. To understand what is meant by "designed experiences," and understand its relationship to nursing education, it is imperative to excavate the theory's foundation in early work on experiential learning.

ROOTS IN DEWEY'S THEORY OF EXPERIENTIAL LEARNING

The theoretical roots of "designed experiences" come out of the experiential learning theory of John Dewey (Squire, 2006). Dewey was a prominent American pragmatist philosopher and educator during the late 19th and early 20th century who brought the experiential theory of learning to prominence in his famous experimental Laboratory School in Chicago (Kolb, Boyatzis, & Mainemelis, 2001). In 1899, Dewey, concerned with the rigid and disciplinary pedagogical model in most American schools, founded the Laboratory School as a philosophy laboratory in which students were taught through methods that acknowledged the unity of knowing and doing. Students, in other words, would learn by doing.

Directed by Dewey while he was chair of the University of Chicago philosophy department, the Laboratory School sought to teach students by connecting what they were learning to real-world, everyday practices, which often took the form of trade skills and crafts. Instead of placing students in highly disciplined classroom environments in which instruction was rote, Dewey sought to use occupational and trade skills to help students connect knowledge learned in-school to the everyday, real world that they encountered outside the classroom. In his popular 1899 book *The School and Society*, which launched progressive education movement on a wide scale in the United States, Dewey articulated the rationale underlying this pedagogical practice:

> In critical moments we realize that the only discipline that stands by us, the only training that becomes intuition, is that got through life itself. That we learn from experience, and from the books and sayings of others *only* as they are related to experience, are not mere phrases. But the school has been so set apart, so isolated from the ordinary conditions and motives of life, that the place that children are sent for discipline is the one place in the world that is most difficult to get experience—the mother of all discipline worth the name.
>
> —*Dewey, 1899, p. 15*

In Dewey's vision, learning and school activities should be joined with the ordinary habits and practices of social and professional life.

The structure of learning and school activity in the Laboratory School reflected Dewey's core belief that learning should be experiential and connected to life in the world. The center of the school was the workshop and the kitchen, in which students not only learned practical and occupational skills, but also learned the underlying foundational principles and subject matter. The occupations, Dewey thought, were powerful learning activities in which learning and doing were united, an opinion he laid out plainly in *School and Society*:

> The great thing to keep in mind, then, regarding the introduction into the school of various forms of active occupation, is that through them the entire spirit of the school is renewed. It has a chance to affiliate itself with life, to become the child's habitat, instead of being only a place to learn lessons having an abstract and remote reference to some possible living to be done in the future. It gets a chance to be a miniature community, an embryonic society.
>
> —*Dewey, 1899, p. 15*

Laboratory School activities relied greatly on professional occupations as an arena for experiential learning. Students learned mathematics through cooking and carpentry, physics through iron-working, and chemistry through cooking. Cooking, in particular, often incorporated multiple subjects, as students measured ingredients for recipes in appropriate amounts (mathematics), learned about the digestion of the food they were cooking (biology), and observed the chemical and physical transformations of the food they were cooking (chemistry). The mere act of cooking boiled eggs at the Laboratory School involved laborious experimentation and temperature-taking with the various temperature states of water (for example cool, simmering and boiling), study of the physical composition of raw eggs and their role in the reproductive cycle of chickens, an examination of the physical changes an egg underwent as it was cooked, and a lesson about the nutritional properties of eggs (Dewey, 1899). In this way, students were taught using the activities and forms of life in which they could participate outside the walls of the school itself, so that learning was connected to their lived experience in the world.

Dewey, it should be noted, was deeply concerned about how to properly structure and introduce a rigorous experiential learning curriculum into schools. Learning in the Laboratory School was not just a free-wheeling affair, but a deliberate and methodical process that taught children how to learn through scientific observation, experimentation and analysis. These techniques were grounded in Dewey's firm belief that active learning must be accompanied by an understanding of the significance of those experiences. Dewey elaborated on this point, writing:

> But observation alone is not enough. We have to understand the *significance* of what we see, hear and touch. This significance consists of the consequences that will result when what is seen is acted upon. A baby may *see* the brightness of a flame and be attracted thereby to reach for it. The significance of the flame is then not its brightness but its power to burn, as the consequence that will result from touching it. We can be aware of consequences only because of previous experiences.
>
> —*Dewey, 1938, p. 68*

In other words, one cannot learn by action alone, but one has to think deeply and critically about the manner and effects of the action to gain understanding from it.

Dewey saw reflection, action and learning as inextricably bound up. Dewey argued that the connection between reflective thought and experience is imperative to the development of understanding:

> Thought or reflection, as we have already seen virtually if not explicitly, is the discernment of a relation between what we try to do and what happens in consequence. No experience having a meaning is possible without some element of thought.
>
> —*Dewey, 1916, p. 169*

The consequences of this position for experiential learning are profound, as they make clear the importance of structured and explicit reflection for good learning to take place. While Dewey laid out an explicit pedagogical structure for using reflection to enhance learning, he also argued that the structure of reflective experience had five general components: (1) confusion; (2) tentative interpretation; (3) an examination and analysis of the problem at hand; (4) a tentative hypothesis; and (5) action upon a firmer hypothesis. Learning from experience, in this account, is about meaningful and structured cycles of action in the world, and organized reflection about that action (Dewey, 1916). Schools and learning institutions, in Dewey's account, should frame their curriculum around this dialogue between action and organized reflection, between doing and critical thought, to facilitate experiential learning.

In both his writings and his work in the laboratory school Dewey laid out a framework for experiential learning that would have far-reaching implications for American education. The focus for Dewey's framework of understanding experiential learning was constructed around three "unities": (1) the unity of abstract knowledge and doing in the real world; (2) the unity of action and reflection; and (3) the unity of the individual with the community. Learners build knowledge through doing, and develop deeper understandings by acting and reflecting on action. They build better understanding of the subject matter and themselves by doing so in a social environment. These three pillars of experiential learning become critically important not only when we turn our attention to understanding digital games and simulations as designed experiences, but also when we focus on understanding the role of reflection and experience in nursing and nurse education.

It is interesting to note that traditional but bygone models of hospital-based nursing education were more closely aligned with Dewey's model of learning by doing, as nursing students were immersed in practice over a 3-year curriculum and gradually became more independent until they had earned their nursing certificate. As nursing education became more academic and less trade or skills based, much of the learning as doing was replaced by traditional academic didactic learning strategies such as lecture. The institutionalization of nursing education occurring within academic institutions was not without merit. The point is that when nursing education moved form the trade method of nursing education to the academic model of education some of the deep experiential opportunities for learning were likely lost.

PROFESSIONAL EDUCATION AND EXPERIENTIAL LEARNING

Over the past two to three decades, the field of nursing has re-engaged Dewey's ideas and nursing scholars have begun to reconceptualize nursing education as an ongoing *reflective practice*, along the lines of the work of Donald Schön (1983) and Patricia Benner (1984). This process of reconceptualization has not just been an adoption of new or renewed pedagogical structures into nursing education, but also a rediscovery of the experiential learning techniques that guided nursing throughout much of the 20th century. This reconceptualization has marked affinities to experiential learning in schools and with games and simulations because of its emphasis on learning through reflection and action.

Responding to what he called a "crisis of the professions" in the early 1980s, MIT education scholar Donald Schön began to call for broader acknowledgement of the power of reflective practice in the professions (Schön, 1983). The "crisis of the professions," Schön argued, was happening because professionals often lacked the ability to deal with real-world practice in a meaningful way. The professions, and professional education, are built upon an epistemological foundation that Schön characterizes as "technical rationality" (Schön, 1983; Shils, 1978). Technical rationality "holds that practitioners are instrumental problem solvers who select technical means best suited to particular purposes" (Schön, 1983, p. 3). To elucidate the relationship between technical rationality and the professions, Schön considers the dilemma of the civil engineer:

> Civil engineers, for example, know how to build roads suited to the conditions of particular sites and specifications. They draw on their

knowledge of soil conditions, materials, and construction technologies to define grades, surfaces, and dimensions. When they must decide what road to build, however, or whether to build it at all, their problem is not solvable by the application of technical knowledge, not even by the sophisticated techniques of a decision theory. They face a complex and ill-defined mélange of topographical, financial, economic, environmental, and political factors.

—Schön, 1983, p. 4

In other words, the difficulty facing professional practitioners, like civil engineers, often lies not in a lack of technical knowledge about a subject, but rather in their ability to understand how to use that technical knowledge in a real-world space. According to Schön, professionals must confront the messiness and complexity of real-world situations, and, out of that complexity, create problem spaces that allow them to use their professional knowledge—selecting out of a complex situation the key contextual details that will allow them to use their professional knowledge in a meaningful way. An inability to confront real-world problems results from a gap between what professionals are taught in their training and what they need to know in the field.

This problem can be especially acute in nursing, where graduate nurses have mastered a huge amount of didactic content but have not yet mastered the rich social context of professional nursing. For example, nursing students and graduate nurses all learn how to interpret medication orders. They know how to give an injection, yet they have little independent problem-solving skills related to when to give the injection, what gauge needle to use, and which injection site is best given the context of any given patient's unique circumstances. In other words, the understanding of several discrete tasks related to medication administration is well understood by the novice, but the totality of those tasks in practice is less understood. Without a situated understanding of the practice of nursing *in situ* the novice may lack the confidence or ability to effectively and efficiently negotiate through the day-to-day intricacies of professional nursing practice.

How then, do professional educators meet the challenges posed by the crisis of the professions? Schön suggests that part of the solution involves seeing professional knowledge and behavior as part of a "professional artistry" in addition to a "professional science". Schön described the different shapes this artistic competency takes:

I have use the term *professional artistry* to refer to the kinds of competence practitioners sometimes display in unique, uncertain and conflicted situations of practice. Note, however, that their artistry is a high-powered, esoteric variant of the more familiar sorts of competence all of us exhibit every day in countless acts of recognition, judgment, and skillful performance. What is striking about both kinds of competence is that they do not depend upon our being able to describe what we know how to do or even entertain in conscious thought the knowledge our actions reveal.

—*Schön, 1983, p. 22*

This *professional artistry*, in other words, is a disposition or sense of comportment toward professional situations that require discernment and acumen. But how can educators help professionals develop this sense of professional artistry? The key to developing professional artistry, according to Schön, is reflection about our actions.

Like Dewey, Schön believes that reflection about our actions is essential to successful learning by doing. And, like Dewey, Schön holds that meaningful reflection involves understanding the consequences of an action. The similarities between the two are striking, and often made explicit by Schön, but differences do persist. Dewey, for example, articulated his view that reflection was essential to meaning-making, writing:

Thought or reflection, as we have already seen virtually if not explicitly, is the discernment of a relation between what we try to do and what happens in consequence. No experience having a meaning is possible without some element of thought.

—*Dewey, 1916, p. 169*

Schön, however, took pains to distinguish between the different modes of thought that accompanied action, arguing that some actions were performed without much thought or reflection:

When we have learned how to do something, we can execute smooth sequences of activity, recognition, decision, and adjustment without having, as we say, to "think about it." On occasion, however, it doesn't [work].

—*Schön, 1983, p. 26*

Schön notes that often an unthinking routine produces an unexpected result—a surprise—and goes on to describe how people grapple with that result:

Something fails to meet our expectation. In an attempt to preserve the constancy of our usual patterns of knowing-in-action, we may respond to surprise by brushing it aside, selectively inattending to the signals that produce it. Or we may respond to it by reflection, and we may do so in one of two ways.

—*Schön, 1983, p. 26*

Reflection and neglect are the two paths that a person can take when they encounter an unpredicted result. Neglect leads inevitably to ignorance of the reason for a surprising result, but reflection can lead a person to learn what, how, or why their action produced an unexpected result.

Reflection can take on different characteristics in different circumstances. For instance, Schön notes that the nature of reflection after an action, and reflection during an action, is actually quite different. He calls these two forms of reflection "reflection-on-action" and "reflection-in-action" respectively. Reflection-on-action takes places either some time after an action or when a person ends an action to stop and think. "Reflection on action," Schön notes "has no direct connection to present action" (1983, p. 26) because it takes places outside of the confines of an action. If we engage in reflection-in action, however, Schön contends that "our thinking serves to reshape what we are doing while we are doing it" (1983, p. 26). Reflection-in-action, Schön argues, gets us to think critically about our strategies of action, understandings of problems and ways of structure of things in the world. Furthermore, reflection-in-action pushes people to experiment ad hoc with different strategies for success in the world. A person who reflects in action is more likely to test out different theories about how to frame and solve a real-world problem, according to Schön. They can try out by "trial and error" new theories about the predicted consequences of their actions, and see the actual consequences in real time. Schön argues that reflection-in-action is distinct from other forms of reflection because it occurs "on the spot" in the middle of an action. As such, reflection-in-action "leads to on-the-spot experiment and further thinking that affects what we do"—an immediate rethinking of our typical strategies of action as they occur. Experts in any given practice are often able to perform reflection-in-action at the same time they are engaged in high-level practice.

Reflection-in-action, however, is in itself a skill. It has to first be taught and learned before it can be performed. How then, can educators and mentors facilitate the learning of reflection-in-action? Schön presents suggestions as to how the learning of reflection in action can be accomplished. Key among them are the notions of *practicum* and *meta-reflection*. Schön describes a good practicum in the following way:

A practicum is a setting designed for the task of learning a practice. In a context that approximates a practice world, students learn by doing, although their doing usually falls short of real-world work. They learn by undertaking projects that simulate and simplify practice; or they take on real-world projects under close supervision. The practicum is a virtual world, relatively free of the pressures, distractions, and risks of the real on, to which, nevertheless, it refers.

—*Schön, 1983, p. 37*

The practicum is a "safe" space in which the learner can begin to master a practice while experiencing lessened consequences than they would find in the real world. In addition, the practicum is a guided space whether a learner can develop their competency in a practice with the aid of feedback from those more knowledgeable. This development occurs not only through reflection-in-action, but also what Schön calls meta-reflection—reflection on reflection-in-action. This reflection on one's reflection can be a powerful tool for reshaping and reimagining future action, which enables a learner to build complex strategies for action and reflection. Schön calls these different levels of reflection a "ladder of reflection" (Schön, 1983, p. 114). This ladder of reflection can include reflections on descriptions of action, reflections on reflections of action, and so on. More abstract levels of reflection allow a student to understand the structure and character of the reflection and knowledgeable action below. According to Schön, the teaching of professionals how to reflect is as much about learning how to reflect-in-action through a practicum, and reflection about that reflection-in-action, as it is acquiring the technical knowledge of that profession.

This chapter would be remiss if Benner's experiential theory of nursing practice, "thinking in action," (Benner, 1984) was not discussed. Benner brings experiential learning theory to nursing education and clinical practice. For Benner, past experience informs the quality of decisions that nurses make in day-to-day practice. As a nurse progresses from novice to expert the quality of clinical decisions made is directly tied to accumulated past experience. An expert clinician should be able to make better decisions and have the ability to process information to inform current practice while clinical scenarios are unfolding in part due to a more meaningful understanding of nursing practice in general and specific understanding of discrete but often repeated patient encounters.

NURSE EDUCATION, EXPERIENTIAL LEARNING AND REFLECTION-IN-ACTION

Schön's experiential learning framework for reflective practice in the professions and Benner's theory of thinking in action have been tremendously influential in contemporary nursing education. In a few short years, they have had a tremendous impact on nursing education, nursing practice and nursing scholarship, as nurses saw reflection as way to connect their "textbook knowledge" with their day-to-day practice. This transformation occurred in part because it connects to a history of nursing education that was largely forgotten when the profession migrated toward a "technical rationalist" model (see Dingwall, Rafferty, & Webster, 1988). But the transformation also occurred because nursing is a field where reflection-in-action and reflection-on-action significantly improve a professional's practice.

The scope and depth of the influence that Schön and Benner's work on reflective practice and experiential learning had on the field of nursing and other clinical professions is clear in scholarship on learning. Literature on nursing and nursing education show the extent of Schön's impact on the field. Atkins & Murphy, writing in the Journal of Advanced Nursing, argued that:

> Recently within nursing there has been an increasing interest in exploring ways in which professionals learn and, in particular, examining the potential of reflection as a learning tool. It has been recognized that there is a need to integrate theory and practice and that reflection may be a tool that can facilitate this process.
>
> —*Atkins & Murphy, 1993, p. 1188*

Two years later, in the same journal, Richardson and Maltby wrote that:

> Since the publication of Schön's seminal book on reflective in 1983, the ability to be able to reflect in and on practice has gained increasing prominence in the nursing profession.
>
> —*Richardson & Maltby, 1995, p. 235*

Schön's work on reflective practice became so prominent in nursing scholarship, in fact, that exploration, examination, and debate about his work became common in the fields' academic journals. This work often focused on: (a) examining the effects of reflection on nursing practice; and (b) understanding how to integrate reflection into nursing education, practice, and mentorship.

Early nursing research on reflective practice focused on understanding the effects of reflective practice on nurses' practice (Powell, 1989; Jarvis, 1992). Powell's (1989) early writing on reflective practice, for example, examined the relationship between experience, knowledge, and reflection-in-action using interview-based techniques. Powell underscored that a nurse's "ward" experience is as important as their mastery of the "technical rationality" underlying their discipline:

> The high scores in the Belief category, and to an extent in the Norm category, suggest that the ward (or community) area is as important as the knowledge base and, as seems apparent from the scores, appears in many cases to provide the knowledge base. The quality of the practice areas is therefore of great importance in the learning of nurses.
>
> —*Powell, 1989, p. 831*

Nurses, Powell argued, learn as much useful knowledge from their experiences in practice and reflection on that practice as they do from their formal education. Powell suggested that formal methods for engaging in joint reflection-in-action on the ward floor would greatly improve nurses' reservoirs of practical knowledge. This area—understanding the role of reflection in informal and formal nursing pedagogy—became a central area of focus for later research.

Other research on reflective practice in nursing focused on understanding how to integrate reflection into both informal and formal learning environments. Atkins & Murphy (1993) made the case for the centrality of reflection in nurse education:

> Practice is central to nursing education. If learning is to occur from practice, then reflection is vital (Benner, 1984). An understanding of the processes of reflection is important, and sufficient attention must be given to developing the skills required to engage in reflection.
> —*Atkins & Murphy, 1993, p. 1191*

Atkins & Murphy (1993) performed a review of the literature on reflective practice and identified five skills associated with "good" reflection: self-awareness, description, critical analysis, synthesis, and evaluation. Burrows (1995) looked at the role of the nurse teacher in promoting critical reflection and reflective practice. Other research has investigated the development of instruments and interventions to promote reflection. Richardson & Maltby (1995) examined the role of diaries in promoting reflection among nursing students, and delineated different "levels" of reflection that could be achieved in diary composition. Other studies often promoted workshops and focus groups as means to achieve reflective practice.

At the same time that scholarship on reflective practice proliferated in nursing, strong criticism of the paradigm emerged. This critical stance derided the lack of theoretical, methodological and pedagogical clarity in research on reflective practice (MacKintosh, 1998). Even among researchers who were doing work on reflective practice, the lack of methodological consistency was often confusing. Atkins and Murphy (1993), for example, cautioned against the use of *post hoc* verbal instruments to measure reflection-in-action:

> Powell's (1989) study of reflection-in-action used by practicing nurses utilizes interview and observation to draw conclusions about practitioners' reflective abilities The study may have failed, however, to identify those practitioners who were reflecting-in-action, but were unable to make verbally explicit the knowledge behind their actions Schön (1983) argues that practitioners may not be able to articulate the knowledge that they use and states explicitly, "reflection-in-action is a process we can deliver without being able to say what we are doing".
> —*Atkins & Murphy, 1993, p. 1191*

Such confusion and inconsistency often drew critiques from nursing researchers, who questioned the value of a teaching and learning framework without definition. MacKintosh (1998) articulated this critique:

It becomes obvious from the evidence above that the use of reflection as a learning strategy or tool for professional development is seriously flawed. Its terms, concepts and framework for implementation lack basic clarity.

—*MacKintosh, 1998, p. 556*

The reliance by reflective practice advocates on workshops and diaries contradicts Schön's focus on learning through reflection-*in*-action, and instead places all emphasis on reflection-*on*-action. As such advocates of reflective practice in nursing seemed to controvert the very tenets of their espoused learning framework (MacKintosh, 1998). In addition, critics often challenged the individualized and unguided nature of reflection in nursing education, arguing that it could lead novice nurses deeper into incorrect practices that could endanger patients and colleagues. Such critiques continue to challenge supporters of reflective practice in nursing education.

These questions about reflective practice and experiential learning in nursing share similarities with challenges that have confronted experiential learning and inquiry-based learning paradigms for years: How do we create learning experiences that ensure the learner builds productive knowledge? How do we help learners reflect *both in and on their actions* in a meaningful way? How can we ensure that learners are building strategic and schematic knowledge about their experiences, and not just falling into routines? These question and others pose substantial problems to the paradigm of reflective practice that should make advocates and practitioners pause and reflect. And these challenges have confronted the experiential learning problem since Dewey's day is one of validity. Learning through experience is a powerful paradigm for building knowledge, but it can sometimes lead learners astray—into incorrect assumptions, unknowing habits or unfounded knowledge. How do educators ensure that experience learning lead to a productive and useful knowledge? How do they give meaningful structure to the powerful buzzing and blooming confusion of learning through experience?

DESIGNED EXPERIENCES IN GAME-BASED LEARNING ENVIRONMENTS

One way to give structure to experiential learning and reflection is by designing the learner's experience in a virtual environment, a method that parallels the "design work" that good educators do in their everyday teaching (Squire, 2006). The strength of the experiential learning paradigm is its ability to foster "deep" knowledge building and reflection in learners. But historically experiential learning has struggled to ensure that learners build the "right" knowledge for any particular domain. Well-crafted game- and simulation-based learning environments solve this puzzle. Good learning games are *designed experiences* because they allow players to learn by acting and experiencing in a well-ordered, problem-solving space. Players of these games and simulations "learn through a grammar of doing and being" (Squire, 2006, p. 19) that is organized around a functional epistemology—a system of knowing that is tied to acting. As such, the designed experiences found in learning games and simulations are rooted in learning through *action* and *reflection*—the two foundations of Schön's reflective practice and Dewey's experiential learning. A player confronts a problem in a digital space, thinks about the solution to the problem, acts to try to solve that problem, receives feedback on the efficacy of that action, and then reflects on that feedback (see Gee, 2005). These action-reflection cycles are pervasive throughout well-designed learning games and simulations.

Good learning games and simulations contain cycles of action-and-reflection that encourage both reflection-in-action and reflection-on-action. Players must often think carefully about their upcoming actions *while* engaged in a game play sequence, and then pause after a game play sequence and re-think their actions based upon the consequences. In this way video game players are forced to not only reflect-in-action during their play, but also stop and reflect-on-action at intervals during the game. Gee (2007) outlines the four-step process of reflection in game play that parellel's Schön's vision of reflective practice:

1. The player must *probe* the virtual world (which involves looking around the current environment, clicking on something, or engaging in a certain action).
2. Based on reflection during and after probing, the player must form a *hypothesis* about what something (a text, object, artifact, event, or action) might mean in a useful situated way.
3. The player *reprobes* the world with that hypothesis in mind, seeing what effect one gets.
4. The player treats this effect as a feedback from the world and accepts or *rethinks* one's original hypothesis. (Gee, 2007, p. 88).

Good games and simulations, in other words, are constructed around these cycles of action and reflection—around thinking, doing and re-thinking. These built-in cycles of activity in games mirror Dewey's (1916) description of learning through experiential reflection: tentative interpretation, analysis and examination, tentative hypothesis, and action upon a firmer hypothesis. Well-designed learning games embody the learning principles of both Dewey and Schön, because the design of problem-solving activities in games require the player to engage in reflection-on-action.

But, as Schön (1983) points out, it is often more difficult for learners to reflect-*in*-action than it is for them to reflect-on-action. This is consistent with Benner's theory of thinking-in-action (1984), because without situated past experience to guide real-time decision making about an unfolding narrative, or in the case of the nursing clinical scenario there may be little or limited understanding to drive reflection-in-action. But the interface and activity structure of games and simulations are often designed to encourage reflection-in-action. The importance of thinking and doing during game play cannot be understated. Players often experience a "flow state" where they concentrate so hard on game play that nothing else seems to matter. (Csikszentmihalyi, 1990; Squire, 2005). Because games encourage reflection-in-action, through flow, and reflection-on-action through feedback, Squire (2005) notes that games have a "flow paradox" in which players both engage in focused activity while pausing to reflect on their experiences in said activity. It is also worthwhile to note that the possibilities for action that the designer gives to the player structures and shapes the flow of game play. Legendary Nintendo game designer Shigeru Miyamoto argued that game design is about building *play-based verbs* that players use to engage in action (Squire, 2006).

The design of play-based verbs is about providing players with avenues for action in an ideological world, and presenting them with problems where they can articulate their mastery of new forms of action. The ongoing, in-the-moment form of thinking-and-doing results as player's consider how to use their virtual abilities in a digital spaces, and are one way among many that games and simulations encourage reflection-in-action and thinking-in-action in a constrained problem solving space. Games and simulations encourage reflection-in-action and thinking-in-action because they are fundamentally built around thinking-and-doing in a virtual space.

The reflection-in-action fostered by learning games and simulations do not occur in a vacuum. Good learning games and simulations structure experiential learning so that action occurs in a well-ordered content domain that is contextually and authentically situated. If we think about game play as a combination of knowing and doing, in a learning game the gist of the knowing part of play is specified before-hand by the game designer, not the player. While a player's decisions can take them and carry them into different trajectories of play (and even into emergent, unintended circumstances), the overarching structure of the player's experience is a product of the fixed design of a knowledge domain.

But well-designed games and simulations are not just scripted, three-dimensional films. They give the player an authentic feeling of experience and empowerment, allowing them to choose from meaningful trajectories of play (DeVane & Squire, 2008). In this way, well-designed games and simulations solve one of the core problems of experiential learning and reflective practice. Learning through experience in games and simulations is not free-form and uncontrolled—allegations that detractors lob at experiential learning pedagogy—but rather well-ordered and specified. At the same time, the experience players have in virtual spaces is immersive, rich and empowering. Learning games and simulations accomplish this feat because of the following characteristics:

1. *Well-ordered problem-solving.* Good learning games and simulations present problems for the player to solve that are appropriate for their skill level. These problems provide the player with a skill-based situation in which they can test their knowledge themselves by engaging in knowledgeable action (Gee, 2007). Problems encourage players to both engage in both knowledgeable action and reflection.
   (a) In the context of nursing education, problem-solving occurring as part of game play should make sense to the learner in the context of nursing practice. For example, checking the "rights" of medication administration should take place before one administers medication, but after receiving and interpreting the order. In this way figuring out the ordering or steps in the process of medication administration is modeled after actual process.
2. *Meaningful goals.* Goals are clearly defined and their rationale articulated by a narrative. Overarching goals, and their narrative rationale, provide players with a *meaningful context* that motivates them to achieve success in problem solving. Upon achievement of goals players are often presented with rewards. Meaningful and authentic contexts for action encourage players to master and reflect on the content they are learning (Squire, 2006).
   (a) For example, nursing students are required to master specific content prior to performing certain skills on actual patients. Students are required to demonstrate a mastery of math skills related to drug calculations before giving medications to actual patients in a real-world supervised clinical environment. Mastery of the math skills related to medication administration is about more than the pen-and-paper test. Demonstrating proficiency in one skill (math) means that the student will be able participate in, and gain experience in new skills (medication administration), whereby clinical experience becomes more robust and interesting. In the same vane, accomplishments demonstrated during game play in the virtual world should lead to opportunity to advance the games narrative.
3. *Possibility spaces.* Many games and simulations present players a multitude of choices; decisions and possibilities for action, letting them formulate an individualized solution to a problem, or custom strategy to accomplish a goal. These virtual worlds are play spaces where players can experiment with their knowledge, beliefs, values and identities (Squire & Jenkins, 2002; Squire, 2007).
   (a) For example, one of the lessons essential to nursing practice focuses on patient confidentiality associated with the Health Insurance Portability

and Accountability Act (HIPAA). Different spaces in the healthcare setting are ideal for different types of action, in this case discussion of private patient information. Students immersed in game play have the ability to engage in conversations in spaces that are both appropriate and inappropriate for discussing patients' private information in the virtual world. Moreover, players are also free to repurpose spaces in-world to meet game and curriculum objectives. In this way if obtaining a confidential patient history is not possible because a spouse or significant other is in the virtual exam room, opportunity still exists (as in the real-world) to use the virtual play space of the created environment to solve the problem at hand.

4. *Feedback and information.* Helpful information encourages players think about and reflect on their action—both during and after the action. This information most often takes the form of feedback and just-in-time information. Feedback is information given to the player after they have completed a problem-solving action or series of actions. Just-in-time information is information that is delivered just as a player confronts a problem where they will use the information. This way of delivering information stimulates reflection-in-action and thinking-in-action. Players understand the relevance of this information to their goals, and reflect on the relevance of the information to their action (Gee, 2005). Both feedback and just-in-time information stimulate players to both reflect-in and reflect-on their action (Steinkuehler & Chmiel, 2006).

   (a) For example, reflection-on-action occurs during game play when learners or students are making decisions based on the results of some earlier action that they have engaged in. When students regularly wash their hands before patient encounters the incidence of hospital-acquired infection goes down. Players have the opportunity, either through self-guided or instructor-guided reflection to reflect on how one facet of practice, hand washing, correlates to best practice.

   (b) Similarly instructors can facilitate thinking-in-action and reflection-in-action through just-in-time information provided to the player in a situationally authentic context. For example, lab values could arrive to drive the objectives of a designed experience by providing cues that reinforce targeted outcome. In this way the lab values provide the impetus for action that will drive not only patient outcome within the context of the game, but will also drive thinking and reflection-in-action, and then future reflection-on action during future game play and during actual real-world clinical encounters.

5. *Empowerment and reward.* Players get a sense of empowerment and accomplishment from their achievements and a real sense of the capacity for their action to have an impact in the virtual space. This sense of empowerment heightens the player's appreciation of their experience (Gee, 2005). The rewards given to players to celebrate their accomplishment heightens

the pleasure players feel in relationship to their achievement. Players are varyingly rewarded with new abilities, goods, *badges*, and decorations that show their accomplishments.

(a) Providing reward for accomplishment is common thread during clinical education. Successful progression through one stage of training leads to more advanced and challenging learning opportunities. This is a common facet of game play that acts to engage the player and maintain their attention. For example, when a learner successfully completes a skill challenge related to IV therapy within the game-based environment, the skill acquisition should help drive the context of the game narrative unfolding for the learner. In other words, because the player now possesses IV skills, the new challenges or problems presenting themselves should serve as a reward for the appropriate application of these skills.

(b) An example of a badge awarded to students marking the successful evolution from student to professional nurse is the transition from a short white coat to a long white coat. This "short coat" versus "long coat" denotes expertise, credibility and membership into the profession.

Experiential learning and reflective practice are fundamentally concerned with bridging the gap between knowing and doing, so that both abstract and practical understandings that a learner builds are fundamentally connected. Well-designed learning games bridge the divide between the context in which doing takes place and the content for learners to know. The design features of games and simulations outlined above serve to connect knowing and doing through play. Through well-structured play, learners confront the connection between knowledge and action. The problem-solving scenarios that players encounter force them to put their knowledge into practice, while feedback and just-in-time information help them build new knowledge by exploring the consequence of application. Learning in well-designed games is fundamentally about learning through performance, about understanding how to use content in a situated context, about reflecting in action. Nursing education is ground zero for experiential learning, because mastery of nursing entails learning the abstract knowledge domain and the ability to practice that knowledge in a professional setting are of the utmost importance.

NURSING EDUCATION AS A DESIGNED EXPERIENCE

Nursing is one of the professional practices that confront stark challenges in the 21st century. Health sciences professionals in Western countries face a rapidly aging population that requires increasing amounts of care. Resources for primary care personnel are scarce even as healthcare costs rise.

To exacerbate this problem, the nursing profession is represented by an aging workforce (Duvall & Andrews, 2010). Further, professional environmental factors and life-style choices often lure younger nurses from the beside and sometimes out of the profession altogether leaving a serious experience gap as older nurses prepare for retirement (Borkowski, Amann, Song, & Weiss, 2007; Cortelyou-Ward, Unruh, & Fottler, 2010; Romano, 2010).

The general use of technology in the health sciences is changing at an ever-increasing rate. Specialization among different disciplines in nursing and other clinicians often lead to the fragmentation of the available technology. Nurses and health sciences professionals are tasked with translating this fragmented, changing technological apparatus into a meaningful and effective system of healthcare. Even so, the evaporating resources available for professional education and clinical learning leave healthcare professionals to cope with changing technological circumstances on their own.

Educational technology in health sciences education has tried to step in and fill the void left by the lack of resources for ongoing education. But its initiatives have focused mostly on "training" rather than educating healthcare professionals to achieve and maintain critical skills and knowledge. Unfortunately, many see training-oriented communication technology as a replacement for a skilled teacher, coach or mentor, and try to use it to "quiz" professionals until they are deemed "taught." In the absence of deliberate instructional design, virtual environments end up transmitting decontextualized skills and behaviors rather than providing context-rich environments where students and professionals can learn to improve their practice. The designed experiences perspective requires educators to think of technology as a tool for creating learning experiences and environments rather than as a replacement for a teacher or mentor. Designed experiences are meaningful, compelling, and information-rich spaces in which learners can experiment, learn, and refine their professional practice rather than a means to train and regiment individuals with unsituated and sometimes irrelevant knowledge and behaviors. The cycles of action and reflection found in designed experiences mirror reflection-in-action and thinking-in-action where nurses and other healthcare professionals could learn in their real-world practice.

DESIGNING EXPERIENCES: MOVING FROM CONTENT TO CONTEXT

Historically designers of digital educational environments have focused on providing well-ordered learning content to users (Squire, 2006). Two outmoded educational models underlie this content-centric paradigm: the "skill-and-drill" and transmission models of learning. Skill-and-drill, or rote, models expect the learner to acquire skills through repetition, often in verbal form. In this paradigm it is important to note that learners are not provided with meaningful contexts where they can practice skills, or well-ordered experiences that build on their prior knowledge. Skill-and-drill paradigms whether found in pen-and-paper format or within digital environments emphasize rote learning, and are popular with advocates of standardized test-driven education. In a similar fashion, the transmission model of learning is focused on displaying information to the learner in a distraction-free and decontextualized digital environment. Because advocates of the transmission model want to reduce the "cognitive load" required to perceive educational content, they design digital software that discourages users from acting with and on information. To this end, the transmission model often strips potentially distracting but important contextual information from the visual interface of learning software. Neither of these approaches allows learners to both build knowledge through experience and engage in action in a meaningful learning context. In doing so, these approaches omit key components of active and relevant learning practice.

Well-designed learning games and simulations provide players with meaningful contexts where they can learn content through experience, experimentation, and world-relevant action (Gee, 2007; Squire, 2006). Clinicians in real-world environments have to learn to quickly *recognize the context* of an evolving diagnosis or patient complaint, and swiftly *enact their knowledge* to solve that problem (Games & Bauman, 2011; Bauman, 2010). The context-rich and experiential affordances of learning games and simulations facilitate the development of these skills. Context, many argue, is a key feature of many games, because the possibilities, aesthetics, and rules that constitute a game context provide avenues for creativity and play. Squire (2006) writes that:

> Many designers have come to see games as vehicles for player expression, thinking of game design as choreographing the rules, representations, and roles for players, in other words the contexts, in which players can generate meaning (LeBlanc, 2005). As such, game designers "write" the parameters for players' experience, and the game experience as such is best described as an interaction between the game designer and player (Robison, 2004).
>
> —*Squire, 2006, p. 21*

We can argue that game play, then, emerges as the "intersection of design constraints with players' intentions" (Squire, 2006, p. 26). Designers of learning games provide the rules, problems, and cues for reflection, and players create an emergent experience out of their intentions, feelings, and activity. Such a combination builds situated and experiential knowledge while allowing players to experiment with their skills in an authentic-feeling safe space for learning. The resultant mixture of well-designed learning and authentic personal experience holds great promise for clinical education in the 21st century.

SUMMARY

In this chapter we described the relationship between learning games and simulations, designed experiences, and reflective practice in nursing. The relationship between these three is both pedagogically closer and historically deeper than one might think. In delineating the contours of this relationship, this chapter has focused on four areas:

1. *Designed experiences with games and simulations.* This chapter described what it means to think of learning games and simulations as designed experiences. It outlined in detail how we understand action and play in digital environments as a designed experience—an experience that emerges from a dialogue between a player's dynamic action and the context of the digital world in which they act.
2. *Designed experiences and experiential learning.* This chapter traced the roots of designed experiences and reflective practice to Dewey's theories of experiential learning, outlining influential historical understandings of what it means to learn through experience. It paid particular attention to how past understandings of contemporary learning are articulated in contemporary design and pedagogy.
3. *Reflective practice, experiential learning and nursing.* This chapter examined the history and importance of reflective practice, an experiential learning paradigm, to nursing education and nursing praxis. It examined both arguments for and against the use of the reflective practice framework in clinical education, and argued that designed experiences enable learner reflection while providing a structured and targeted learning experience.
4. *Learning in designed experiences.* This chapter outlined how learning actually occurs in the "designed experience" of learning games and simulations. It described and explicated the features of games that immerse players in meaningful learning contexts, ranging from problem-solving and just-in-time feedback to feelings of empowerment and possibility. It argued that designed experiences allow educators to structure the content domain of experiential learning activities.

REFERENCES

Atkins, S., & Murphy, K. (1993). Reflection: A review of the literature. *Journal of Advanced Nursing, 18*(8), 1188–1192.

Barab, S., & Duffy, T. (2000). From practice fields to communities of practice. *Theoretical foundations of learning environments, 1*, 25–55.

Bauman, E. (2007). High fidelity simulation in healthcare. Ph.D. dissertation, The University of Wisconsin – Madison, United States. Dissertations & Theses @ CIC

Institutions database. (Publication no. AAT 3294196 ISBN: 9780549383109 Pro-Quest document ID: 1453230861)

Bauman, E. (2010). Virtual reality and game-based clinical education. In K. Gaberson, & M. Oermann (Eds.), *Clinical teaching strategies in nursing* (3rd ed., pp. 183–212). New York: Springer.

Benner, P. (1984). *From novice to expert: Excellence and power in clinical nursing practice.* Menlo Park, CA: Addison-Wesley.

Borkowski, N., Amann, R., Song, S. H., & Weiss, C. (2007). Nurses' intent to leave the profession: Issues related to gender, ethnicity and educational level. *Health Care Management Review, 32*(2), 160–167.

Burrows, D. E. (1995). The nurse teacher's role in the promotion of reflective practice. *Nurse Education Today, 15*(5), 346–350.

Campbell, S. H., & Daley, K. M. (2009). Simulation scenarios for nurse educators: Making it real. New York: Springer Publishing Company.

Cortelyou-Ward, K. H., Unruh, L., & Fottler, M. D. (2010). The effect of work environment on intent to leave the nursing profession: A case study of beside nursing in rural Florida. *Health Services Management Research, 23*(4), 185–192.

Csikszentmihalyi, M. (1990). Flow: The psychology of optimal experience. New York: Harper & Row.

Dewey, J. (1899). *The school and society: Being three lectures by John Dewey.* Chicago: University of Chicago Press.

Dewey, J. (1902). *The child and the curriculum.* Chicago: University of Chicago Press.

Dewey, J. (1916). *Democracy and education.* New York: MacMillan Company.

Dewey, J. (1926). *Democracy and education.* Raleigh, NC: Hayes Barton Press.

Dewey, J. (1938). *Experience and education.* New York: MacMillan Company.

DeVane, B., & Squire, K. (2008). The meaning of race and violence in grand theft auto. *Games and Culture, 3*(3–4), 264–285.

DeVane, B., Durga, S., & Squire, K. (2010). "Economists Who Think Like Ecologists": Reframing systems thinking in games for learning. *E-Learning and Digital Media, 7*(1), 3–20.

DeVita, M. (2005). Organizational factors affect human resuscitation: The role of simulation in resuscitation research. *Critical Care Medicine, 33*(5), 1150–1151.

Dingwall, R., Rafferty, A. M., & Webster, C. (1988). *An introduction to the social history of nursing.* London: Routledge.

Duvall, J. J., & Andrews, D. R. (2010). Using a structured review of the literature to identify key factors with the current nursing shortage. *Journal of Professional Nursing, 26*(5), 309–317.

Ericsson, K. A., Krampe, R. T., & Tesch-Römer, C. (1993). The role of deliberate practice in the acquisition of expert performance. *Psychological review, 100*(3), 363.

Flanagan, B., Nestel, D., & Joseph, M. (2004). Making patient safety the focus: Crisis resource management in the undergraduate curriculum. *Medical Education, 38*(1), 56–66.

Friedrich, M. J. (2002). Practice makes perfect: Risk-free medical training with patient simulators. *Jama, 288*(22), 2808, 2811–2812.

Gaba, D. M. (2004). The future vision of simulation in health care. *Quality and Safety in Health Care, 13*(Suppl. 1), 2–10.

Gaba, D. M., Howard, S. K., Fish, K., Smith, B., & Sowb, Y. (2001). Simulation-based training in anesthesia crisis resource management (ACRM): A decade of experience. *Simulation & Gaming, 32*(2), 175–193.

Games, I. A., & Bauman, E. B. (2011) Virtual worlds: An environment for cultural sensitivity education in the health sciences. *International Journal of Web Based Communities*, 7(2), 189–205, doi: 10.1504/IJWBC.2011.039510.

Gee, J. P. (2003). *What videogames have to teach us about learning and literacy.* New York, NY: Palgrave-McMillan.

Gee, J. (2005). Learning by design: Good video games as learning machines. *E-Learning, 2*(1), 5–16.

Gee, J. (2007). Learning and games. *The ecology of games*, The John D. and Catherine T. MacArthur Foundation Series on Digital Media and Learning (pp. 21–40).

Gee, J. P. (2007). *What video games gave to tTeach us about learning and literacy* (2nd ed.). New York: Palgrave Macmillan.

Gladwell, M. (2008). *Outliers: The story of success*. New York, NY: Little, Brown and Company.

Gordon, J. A., Oriol, N. E., & Cooper, J. B. (2004). Bringing good teaching cases "to life": A simulator-based medical education service. *Academic Medicine, 79*(1), 23–27.

Hammond, J. (2004). Simulation in critical care and trauma education and training. *Current Opinion Critical Care, 10*(5), 325–329.

Helmreich, R. L. (2000). On error management: Lessons from aviation. *British Medical Journal, 320*(7237), 781–785.

Jarvis, P. (1992). Reflective practice and nursing. *Nurse Education Today, 12*(3), 174–181.

Jasper, M. (2003). *Beginning reflective practice*. Cheltenham: Nelson Thornes.

Kolb, D. A., Boyatzis, R. E., & Mainemelis, C. (2001). Experiential learning theory. Previous research and new directions. In R. J. Sternberg & L. Zhang (Eds.), *Perspectives on thinking, learning, and cognitive style: The educational psychology series* (pp. 227–247). Mahwah, NJ: Erlbaum.

Lane, J. L., Slavin, S., & Ziv, A. (2001). Simulation in medical education: A review. *Simulation & Gaming, 32*(3), 297–314.

Larew, C., Lessans, S., Spunt, D., Foster, D., & Covington, B. (2006). Innovations in clinical simulation: Application of benner's theory in an interactive patients care simulation. *Nursing Education Perspectives, 27*(1), 16–21.

LeBlanc, M. (2005). Tools for creating dramatic game dynamics. In K. Salen & E. Zimmerman (Eds.), *Thegamedesign reader: Arules of play anthology* (pp. 438–459). Cambridge, MA: MIT Press.

Lee, S. K., Pardo, M., Gaba, D., Sowb, Y., Dicker, R., Straus, E. M. et al. (2003). Trauma assessment training with a patient simulator: A prospective, randomized study. *Journal of Trauma Injury Infection and Critical Care, 55*, 651–657.

Mackintosh, C. (1998). Reflection: A flawed strategy forthe nursing profession. *Nurse Education Today, 18*(7), 553–557.

McLellan, B. A. (1999). Early experience with simulated trauma resuscitation. *Canadian Journal of Surgery, 42*(3), 205–210.

Powell, J. H. (1989). The reflective practitioner in nursing. *Journal of Advanced Nursing, 14*(10), 824–832.

Richardson, G., & Maltby, H. (1995). Reflection on practice: Enhancing student learning. *Journal of Advanced Nursing, 22*(2), 235-242.

Robison, A. (2004). *The "internal design grammar" of video games.* Paper presented at the annual meeting of the American Educational Research Association, San Diego, CA.

Romano, A. (2010). The great divide: The culture of beside nurses and nurse managers. *Nurse Leader, 7*(5), 47-50.

Schön, D. A. (1983). *The reflective practitioner: How professionals think in action.* New York: Basic Books.

Shapiro, M. J., & Simmons, W. (2002). High fidelity medical simulation: A new paradigm in medical education. *Medicine & Health, Rhode Island, 85*(10), 316-317.

Shils, E. (1978). The order of learning in the United States from 1865 to 1920: The ascendancy of the universities. *Minerva, 16*(2), 159-195.

Skinner, B. F. (1960). Teaching machines. *The Review of Economics and Statistics, 42*(3 Part 2), 189-191

Squire, K. D. (2005). Educating the fighter: Buttonmashing, seeing, being. *On the Horizon, 13*(2), 75-88.

Squire, K. D. (2006). From content to context: Videogames as designed experience. *Educational Researcher, 35*(8), 19-29.

Squire, K. D. (2007). Open-ended video games: A model for developing learning for the interactive age. In K. Salen (Ed.), *The ecology of games*, The John D. and Catherine T. MacArthur Foundation series on digital media and learning (pp. 167-198). Cambridge: MIT Press.

Squire, K. D., DeVane, B., & Durga, S. (2008). Designing centers of expertise for academic learning through video games. *Theory Into Practice, 47*(3), 240-251.

Squire, K. D., & Jenkins, H. (2002). The art of contested spaces. In L. King, & C. Bain (Eds.), *Game on* (pp. 62-75). London: Barbarican.

Steinkuehler, C., & Chmiel, M. (2006). Fostering scientific habits of mind in the context of online play (pp. 723-729). Presented at the Proceedings of the 7th international conference on Learning sciences, International Society of the Learning Sciences.

Ziv, A., Wolpe, P. R., Small, S. D., & Glick, S. (2003). Simulation-based medical education: An ethical imperative. *Academic Medicine, 78*(8), 783-788.

II

Using Technology and Game-Based Learning in Your Curriculum and in Your "Classroom"

4

Preparing Faculty and Students for Game-Based and Virtual Learning Spaces

ERIC B. BAUMAN

INTRODUCTION

Game-based learning and simulation tools represent a relatively new space within nursing education and other clinical disciplines. Educators must be well oriented to technology that supports game-based learning tools and virtual spaces to maximize the usefulness of this new technology. Additionally, it is essential for administration to support faculty and instructors to help ensure that meaningful learning takes place when teaching in these new and often novel spaces. Educators must sufficiently orient students to support any learning space to decrease anxiety and promote learning experiences as safe and positive. This is particularly critical when the learning space being introduced represents a new experience for learners. Providing preparatory, ongoing, and expert technical support to meet both teachers' and learners' needs is essential to the teaching (faculty or instructor) and the learning (student) experience. To this end, faculty, staff, and students alike must clearly understand tutorials detailing *environmental fidelity* and environment or platform limitations.

Communicating expectations associated with curriculum objectives that occur in different types of learning spaces is not novel. For example, we expect students to behave in different prescribed ways in the classroom, in the nursing lab, and in actual clinical environments. Similarly, we explain and contrast the limitations of deliberate practice taking place in a fixed simulation lab versus how those same skills will be demonstrated in a supervised real-world clinical environment.

Similarly, it is important for faculty to convey their expectations of students who are engaging a virtual or game-based learning environment. By way of example, those teachers familiar with online teaching and learning platforms understand the challenges associated with getting students to interact in a meaningful way in the absence of togetherness found in a traditional classroom. Students benefit from interaction that allows for informal communication before, after, and often during a class. When teachers seek group work or peer-to-peer problem solving within online courses it often requires coaxing or a tangible reward. In other words, it is paramount that teachers communicate course and lesson objectives when learner engagement is not necessarily reinforced by regular face-to-face, student-to-teacher communication (Tyczkowski, Bauman, Gallagher-Lepak, Vandenhouten, & Resop Reilly, in press).

FACULTY READINESS AND DEVELOPMENT FOR TECHNOLOGY INTEGRATION

Faculty Buy-In and Engagement

We have and will continue to stress the importance of choosing technology that supports curriculum objectives and student needs as a common thread throughout this book. This said, without buy-in from faculty, engaging technology that represents a change in educational delivery and what counts for acceptable pedagogy, let alone a paradigm shift in the digital millennia, often results in push back and disenfranchisement from faculty.

For example, a well-established Midwest 2-year technical college system made the requirement that all curricula, related objectives, and assessment guidelines be made available online to all students and the general public. The goal of this decision was to better prepare students for enrollment, the courses being taught, and to establish consistency among the same courses often being taught across the numerous campuses throughout the state. However, scant resources were made available to assist faculty in this process. The process followed an online template and interface to be completed by faculty and support staff. Unfortunately, faculty had little input into the project itself or the project implementation process. Further, little, if any training was made available for faculty to achieve proficiency, let alone expertise in this process. In short, a process designed to leverage technology to improve learner experience failed to engage school faculty. In the end, many questioned whether or not students benefited from the project at all.

In another example, when a well-known Midwest nursing school that included both an undergraduate baccalaureate program and a graduate program (MS and PhD) embraced online learning, they began by integrating course materials using the university's online course template. A number of courses began to alternate between face-to-face course delivery and online delivery. This decision occurred with little input from faculty. The challenges for faculty included the effort associated with learning to use the online course template and the redesign of face-to-face courses for the online environment at a time when online teaching was still relatively novel. In short, in order for faculty to be successful in this task, they had to learn a new technology and emerging pedagogy associated with it.

Those inexperienced with online or distance learning sometimes attempt to replicate the classroom experience as closely as possible through digital reproduction of classroom lectures or reformatting existing course content. Simply importing face-to-face lesson plans into a digital medium rarely if ever provides a positive experience for teachers or learners (Tyczkowski et al. in press). In the above example, even courses that continued to be taught face-to-face began to use online templates to support course materials. These courses also encountered challenges. Unfortunately the online interface for the courses was often fraught with insufficient student and faculty information technology (IT) and instructional design (ID) support. Making a course available online may in theory increase availability to course resources and increase the number of students who are able to take the course, but it does not necessarily make the course more convenient, or better. A quality online course is a blend of a knowledgeable, skilled facilitator (instructor); relevant, current course materials; and a technically sound, accessible, well-designed course with activities and assessments aligned to learning objectives. In other words, a blend of IT, ID, and instructor expertise.

As discussed in Chapter 1, mannikin-based simulation began making its appearance in earnest in the context of clinical education in the 1960s with the advent of the CPR mannikin invented by Norwegian toymaker Asmund Laerdal (Grenvik & Schaefer, 2004) and the introduction of Harvey, a complex mannikin used to teach cardiac diagnostic skills (Cooper & Taqueti, 2004). Other types of simulators for clinical education followed and continue to be introduced today (Bauman, 2007). This history illustrates that the learning curve for faculty and instructors related to the introduction of new technology integration for nursing and other curricula has always existed and will continue to exist.

Each iteration of technology that faculty encounter represents and continues to pose a relatively steep learning curve. From the simple airway and CPR mannikins of the past, to today's complex high-fidelity mannikin simulators of and virtual and game-based learning environments, the learning curve is both steep and a function of users current and past experience. In other words, the challenge associated with learning to use new technology may not be, and likely is not, a function of poor technology design, but rather, a generational divide that often exists among new, often younger faculty and senior faculty. Further, this divide certainly exists among most students and even the youngest faculty. Prensky (2001, 2010) discusses the implications of this generational divide by referring to the net (as in Internet) or digital generation as *digital natives* and those of us who have adopted digital technology as adults or later in life as *digital immigrants*.

Today's (traditional) students are all *digital natives;* they are fluent in the language of the digital environment. They possess an innate sense of media literacy. They are far more comfortable with new and emerging technology than their faculty, in part because the rapid advancement of digital technology has always been persistent as part of their social and educational experience. Many faculty, as digital immigrants, must learn to navigate, communicate, and leverage the digital age. Not unlike traditional immigrants, digital immigrants adapt to their new environments with varying levels of success and comfort. Most immigrants retain some historical grounding. Digital immigrants remember the way it used to be, and to some degree the negotiation of change and history will frame the digital immigrants' perceptions of new technology and their attempts at assimilation into the digital landscape (Prensky, 2001, 2010).

The goals of technology integration should always focus on leveraging the new technology for the benefit of curriculum objectives, achievement, and enhanced learning or student experience. In order to ensure that technology meets these goals it is essential to support faculty in ways that, at a minimum, ensure their buy-in with the hope of fostering champions who embrace the new technology and related pedagogy.

Faculty engagement is also supported by including them as major stakeholders from the beginning of the technology integration process including conceptualization, curriculum change or development, implementation, and outcome evaluation (Aleckson & Ralston-Berg, 2011). Engaging faculty in this way vests them in the outcome. Including faculty throughout the technology acquisition and implementation process informs them about the effort, capital, and commitment that is required to prepare them and others to leverage technology in a way that supports program objectives. Marshaling faculty as vested stakeholders is particularly important when embracing game-based learning taking place in virtual environments, because misunderstanding of the pedagogy supporting this technology and a host of stereotypes often accompany this medium (Shaffer, Squire, Halverson, & Gee, 2005; Squire, 2006; Williams, Yee, & Caplan, 2008).

In order to overcome misunderstanding and stereotyping related to game-based learning, administrators and faculty should be provided with scholarly material that informs them from the scientific and research perspective (Aleckson & Ralston-Berg, 2011). Whether administrators are informing faculty or faculty are informing administrators is irrelevant. Those introducing and advocating game-based learning strategies should be prepared to make an academic and scholarly case for their integration into existing and new curricula.

Some refer to game-based learning as serious gaming. Some scholars and teachers in the academic environment have made the assertion that for serious gaming to be effective it cannot be fun. From this perspective fun need not and should not be included in learning processes that support knowledge transfer or acquisition that leads to effective clinical decision making. This perspective or stereotype is not supported in this text nor among scholars in the game-based learning movement; nevertheless, it is a perspective. Historically, learning is associated with work, while games are associated with fun. Yet the very nature of play requires learning to take place. Games "... trigger deep learning that is itself part and parcel of the fun. It is what makes good games deep." (Gee, 2004, p. 23). Serious games are becoming widely available, and as the audience grows serious games are beginning to gain acceptance as viable teaching tools to promote behavioral change and target important learning objectives (Lieberman, 2009).

Other stereotypes or perspectives do not see the utility in video games for adult education, let alone clinical education. Instead video games are seen as child's play with no place in professional or clinical education. Again, the contributing authors of this text do not support this position nor is this position supported by the many scholars in the game-based learning movement. In fact, the largest growing demographic of video game players is found in the adult population. The majority of America's adults play video games (53%). One in five adults play video games daily or almost every day (Lenhart, Jones, & Mcgill, 2008; Williams, Martins, Conslavo, & Ivory, 2009). According to the Entertainment Software Association (http://www.theesa.com/facts/gameplayer.asp), adult women are the fastest growing population of game players, and 55% of all game players play on a mobile device.

Further, others are biased by their perception and the commonly held stereotype that violence permeates most or all of the video game industry and that violence occurring in the narrative of commercial video games has somehow obviated the potential of game-based learning and learning taking place in virtual environments in general. This is a largely unsupported assumption, even though the topic of violence found in commercial video games remains politically charged (Greenfield, 2010; Squire, 2003). Research in the area of violence, aggression, and video games largely focuses on children, not adult populations, or adult populations engaging in clinical or professional education. Further, adult learners are more self-motivated with higher levels of autonomy and cognitive experience than their primary and secondary education counterparts. In this sense, enrolled nursing students and other clinical health sciences students are already self-selecting and have been screened into programs based on academic performance and vetted assumptions about their character and social as well as cultural mores.

STRATEGIES FOR SUCCESSFUL INTEGRATION OF GAME-BASED LEARNING: EXISTING EXPERTS

Champions supporting new and novel technology for nursing education are essential to successful integration. One or two champions within a school or department are usually easy to find because they are often self-selecting and in many cases responsible for the introduction or proposed introduction of new and novel technology-based tools for instruction. Engaging other faculty members can be more difficult. However, if educators solicit and nurture strategic champions among leadership and administration, the process of faculty engagement, even among the reluctant is more likely. When leadership identifies with and supports change, it provides strategy, importance, and legitimacy among stakeholders throughout the institution. It sends the message that it is OK and in the best interest of faculty to take an interest in whatever change is being proposed. In this case, the adoption of game-based learning and novel or different pedagogy is best suited to support and integrate this style of learning throughout the curriculum.

Yet some will persist in their assumption that learning processes tailored for clinical education cannot be fun if they are to be effective in teaching students how to make critical clinical life and death decisions. As discussed earlier in this chapter, this perspective or stereotype is not supported in the literature. Rather, increasingly more scholarly literature supports the importance of player experience to promote behavioral change (Baranowski, Buday, Thompson, & Baranowski, 2008). In other words positive, enjoyable, or fun experiences can be transformative and translational.

A body of research is beginning to develop that supports the utility of video games for adult education for professional and clinical training (Hayes, 2005; Telner et al., 2010). Unfortunately, despite evidence to the contrary, some clinical educators continue to see video games as child's play with no place in professional and clinical education, even as game-based learning for clinical and professional education continues to glean impressive national attention, including from the Robert Wood Johnson Foundation (Kron, Gjerde, Sen, & Fetters, 2010). Recall, as discussed earlier in this chapter, that the largest growing demographics of video game players are found among the adult population (Lenhart et al., 2008; www.theesa.com/facts/gameplayer. asp). Further, there is currently a senior policy analyst for the Office of Science and Technology within the United States Executive Office of the President who advises on the role of technology, including video games and learning. It is little surprise that clinical educators are exploring games to engage learners and meet program objectives.

DEVELOPING EXPERTISE

While one or two experts supporting technology such as game-based learning often exist in schools and programs hoping to integrate this style of learning throughout the curriculum, it is important to develop additional expertise as well. When the institutional expectation is that instructors and faculty will integrate new and innovative teaching strategies and technology, it is important that all instructors develop some level of familiarity and comfort with the technology itself and supporting pedagogy.

Existing experts should be encouraged and rewarded for mentoring colleagues in their use of simulation and game-based learning. Further, resources should be allocated to develop expertise through professional development opportunities. Examples of professional development opportunities include joining academic and professional organizations that specifically support simulation and game-based learning. Three examples of such organizations include the Society for Simulation in Healthcare (SSH), the International Nursing Association for Clinical Simulation and Learning (INACSL), and Games for Health (G4H).

SSH (www.ssih.org) was founded in 2004 and is a multiprofessional, multidiscipline organization that supports healthcare education and research using simulation. In the last several years, SSH has expanded to include a special interest group specific to serious games and virtual environments and how these tools can be used to support clinical education and research. SSH specifically supports the development of health sciences curriculum and analysis of educational and clinical outcomes. SSH also supports the academic journal *Simulation in Healthcare* (Wolters Kluwer/Lippincott Williams & Wilkins) and the annual International Meeting for Healthcare (IMSH) which garners well over 3,000 attendees per year.

The International Nursing Association for Clinical Simulation and Learning (INACSL, www.inacsl.org), a nursing-specific organization, also supports and promotes research and education methodologies for simulation-based and other learning environments. Additionally, INACSL supports an academic journal, *Clinical Simulation in Nursing* (Elsevier) and the Annual International Nursing Simulation/Learning Resource Center Conference.

In addition to these two organizations and their conferences and academic journals, Games for Health (www.gamesforhealth.org/), a project supported by the Robert Wood Johnson Foundation, also brings an important perspective to the discussion of games and education in healthcare. The Games for Health project supports an annual conference in the United States and facilitates learning workshops internationally. In general, Games for Health provides the patient-education perspective on game-based learning. Games for Health also encourages collaboration among academics and industry to promote research and development of the game-based learning movement specific to healthcare.

In addition, to the above-mentioned organizations and journals, 2011 saw the debut of the academic *Games for Health* journal (Mary Ann Liebert, Inc., publisher). This publication is unrelated to the Games for Health organization and conference. Within the general scope of games and simulation but aside from healthcare-specific journals, there are a variety of other academic journals that focus on the genre of game-based learning and simulation. The point is that the pedagogy of game-based learning is relatively new to healthcare, but is not new to other academic disciplines. Below is a list of academic publications related to games and simulation that are not exclusive to healthcare.

- *Computer Game Education Review*, AK PETERS, LTD (http://cger.akpeters.com/)
- *Edudamos: Journal for Computer Game Culture*, Open Journal System/ Public Knowledge Project (www.eludamos.org)

- *Games Studies: The International Journal of Computer Game Research*, The Swedish, Research Council, The Joint Committee for Nordic Research Councils for the Humanities and Social Sciences. IT University of Copenhagen, Lund University (http://gamestudies.org)
- *Games*, MDPI Publishing (www.mdpi.com/journal/games)
- *Games and Culture*, Sage Publications (http://gac.sagepub.com/)
- *Simulation*, Sage Publications (http://sim.sagepub.com/)
- *Simulation & Gaming*, Sage Publications (http://sag.sagepub.com/)
- *International Journal of Intelligent Games and Simulation*, University of Wolverhampton UK (www.scit.wlv.ac.uk/~cm1822/ijigs11.htm)
- *International Journal of Web Based Communities*, InderScience Publishers (http://www.inderscience.com/browse/index.php?journalCODE=ijwbc)
- *International Journal of Gaming and Computer-Mediated Simulations*, IGI Global (www.igi-global.com/journal/international-journal-gaming-computer-mediated/1125)
- *Journal of Virtual Worlds Research*, Virtual Worlds Institute, Inc (http://jvwresearch.org/)
- *Journal of Simulation*, Palgrave McMillan (www.palgrave-journals.com/jos/index.html)
- *Simulation Modelling Practice and Theory*, Elsevier (www.journals.elsevier.com/simulation-modelling-practice-and-theory/)

Expertise in game-based learning is also acquired through research. While this will be explicitly discussed in Chapter 9, it is important to emphasize that all programs should engage in the research process at some level. Any time a new pedagogy is introduced, or for that matter a change in curriculum occurs, it is important to evaluate the change for effectiveness in terms of student experience and whether or not the change has advanced and met program goals and objectives. This sort of evaluation and research should not be seen as solely the job of large research institutions and universities. Teachers and administrators at all levels must have assurance that their curriculum is effective and meeting the needs and goals of their learners. Engaging in research produces expertise. Engaging in clinical research establishes best practices and drives positive patient outcomes. Similarly, engaging in educational research promotes best practices that drive educational outcomes and positive student experiences. The scientific process is inherently educational and promotes not only discrete expertise in the subject matter being investigated, but also promotes a sense of lifelong learning.

LEARNING TO TEACH AS A FACILITATOR AND GUIDE

Teaching with simulation and game-based learning requires the instructor to see teaching from a new perspective. In this style of learning the teachers must avoid seeing students as empty vessels to be filled with domain-specific knowledge. Instead, in the created learning environments found among simu-lation and game-based learning, teachers design experiences that target specific lessons and objectives (Bauman, 2010; Squire, 2006). The teacher then acts as a guide providing just-in-time information to direct learning and keep students on track. The designed experience can take place in advance of, or concurrent with, student immersion in the environment. Different types of programming and control interfaces allow for varying levels of real-time instructor control. At the conclusion of the learning scenario the instruc-tional faculty and staff provide a learner-centered but guided debriefing of learner performance.

During the learning scenario or game-play, students have the opportunity to engage in reflection-in-action (Schön, 1983), and thinking-in-action (Benner, 1984). At the conclusion of game play, during the instructor-guided debriefing, students begin the reflective process of reflection-on-action (Schön, 1983). The reflection-on-action is essential for beginning and novice students because they will lack the experiential expertise to engage in situated in-action reflection.

For example, nursing students who are for the first time encountering a respiratory emergency likely will have difficulty recognizing the connection between bradycardia and hypoxia. This does not necessarily indicate that these students have not mastered the didactic physiologic content related to hypoxia, but rather may mean that they have no situated context to recognize the presenting signs and symptoms, or patterns associated with hypoxia. Until this experience has occurred, the students have no past-situated cognitive experience to guide them in the moment or during future similar patient encounters. The ability to recognize patterns within specific situational context allows experts to make accurate decisions more quickly and with a higher degree of accuracy than novices (Gee, 2003). Lessons designed for virtual learning environments are more successful when instructional designers and teachers situate objectives within the professional context that will eventually recall them during future clinical practice (Gisondi, Smith-Coggins, Harter, Soltysik, & Yarnold, 2004). The term *situated* or *situated context* simply refers to experiences that are seen as a map to authentic pro-fessional practice. In other words, situated experiences are those experiences that also exist within the practice being modeled—in the context of this text, nursing or another clinical practice.

The nature and quality of a post-encounter debriefing will assist with student acceptance of simulation and game-based learning. It helps build a rich, reflective experience to guide future problem solving. The role of the instructor during debriefing is to guide students to epiphanies, rather than telling students what they did correctly or wrong. This does not mean that no instructor-based feedback occurs. Instructors continue to provide and reinforce content through clinical expertise. For example, based on the above example of how hypoxia causes bradycardia in respiratory emergencies, the teacher should avoid telling students that they failed to rescue the patient because they entirely missed the hypoxia and perhaps this occurred because students did not complete the assigned readings. A facilitated debriefing approach would ask the students how they felt the scenario unfolded. As needed, during the debriefing facilitators would ask why students felt the patient became bradycardic. This would probably facilitate a situated discussion about applied respiratory and cardiac physiology, the likely objective of the entire designed experience occurring within the simulation or game-play. If students do not come to the epiphany, instructors are still free to move them toward lesson objectives. This style of teaching helps teachers to understand why students sometimes get to very dangerous clinical places for very good reasons.

Finally, teaching faculty must understand that the learning taking place using designed experiences has the potential to evoke strong emotional responses among students. Guided debriefing sessions must diffuse and mitigate these emotional responses to ensure the psychological safety of students. The debriefing also provides the important opportunity for faculty to set the record straight when or if deception has been used to drive the psychological fidelity of the learning experience (Bauman, 2007; Thiagarajan, 1992).

IMPORTANCE OF STUDENT ORIENTATION AND ASSESSMENT OF LEARNER READINESS FOR TECHNOLOGY: SETTING THE TONE

While students come to colleges and schools expecting some level of technology integration and they will likely have heard about the merits and "coolness" of simulation from more senior students, they may not possess the "learning is fun" mindset. The authors of this textbook accept and promote game-based learning and believe that learning that is situated, engaging, and interactive is inherently more fun than other more static methods of knowledge transfer. We also believe evidence is mounting to support the idea that simulation and game-based learning can be effective. This said, not all of our colleagues have come to appreciate this point of view. Further, not all students will initially embrace this style of learning, particularly if it does not meet their initial expectation of clinical education and training.

A good segue into multimedia game-based learning is to orient and initiate students with hands-on, face-to-face game play. A wide variety of face-to-face, hands-on games focusing on leadership and critical thinking have been used primarily in the area of adult education and business management. There are a variety of resources available to introduce instructors to face-to-face games that can be incorporated into lesson plans. Sivasailam Thiagarajan, one of the pioneers in game-based learning, maintains a website with a number of free training games and resources (www.thiagi.com). Many of the face-to-face games and exercises envisioned for adult education and business management can easily be reframed to emphasize objectives found in clinical education.

Reframing the mindset of learning to represent a fun and engaging experience before immersing your students into a technologically complex environment will help to achieve learner buy-in for game-based pedagogies. As with any game-based learning experience, games should be chosen to reinforce course content and objectives, whether the games being incorporated into the lesson plan are low-tech face-to-face games or existing in created environments of simulation laboratories or virtual reality.

STUDENT ORIENTATION AND LEARNER READINESS

Students must be oriented to all learning spaces whether they occur in the real world or in virtual spaces. Students need to be oriented to new real-world clinical environments in order to understand the environment they are working in and come to an understanding of what clinical performance benchmarks are expected of them. Even within the same hospital, different units have various nuances that students and even new hires to the unit must understand in order to be successful. Orientation to new learning or work spaces takes place on two levels. Organizations and hospitals establish practice guidelines that are disseminated to various nursing units and practice settings. These practice settings interpret organizational guidelines with some degree of variance. It is idealistic to assume that all emergency departments, obstetrical units, or pediatric clinics, even if they exist within the same organization, will have identical practice expectations based on accepted organizational policy. Students in all environments must understand and be oriented to each practice environment and variations and nuances that exist in these discrete environments.

The official and anecdotal paradigm exists when students are expected to perform in simulation and game-based learning environments as well. Different teaching faculty and staff will have different performance expectations of students even when using the same environment. However, the virtual or game-based environments and even mannikin-based simulation laboratories share some additional characteristics that make student orientation to the learning space particularly salient.

Students often need guidance in understanding what is and is not possible in mannikin-based simulation laboratories. Without orientation, students will not know the limitations of the mannikin itself or the equipment found in the laboratory. Further, because we are rarely testing a student's knowledge of where something is kept in the laboratory or how to turn on or use a piece of equipment, it is unreasonable to expect that learners will understand the nuances and exceptions to standard practice that exist in created environments.

The challenge of knowing what is possible and what is not possible in the virtual environment is exacerbated without instructor and self-guided orientation. Providing haptic or hands-on feedback in virtual environments continues to be a real challenge. Completing hands-on skills often requires some sort of "work-around" or "magic." Students must understand the "magic." For example, placing an IV, changing a dressing, or hand washing will be represented in virtual spaces but will occur as a visual representation of an inherently haptic task.

Easter eggs are novel facets of the environment that provide useful information, tangible reward, or entertainment value of some kind. This variable of game play engages and vests players in the game and in the virtual world itself (Bauman, 2010). Easter eggs encourage discovery and exploration of the environment. In this way, they promote orientation to the environment while leaving "no stone unturned."

Also, because the virtual space is not physical, the process of discovery and exploration may not be as intuitive to all learners. This said, processes like discovery and exploration that leave no stone unturned are incredibly powerful learning and teaching tools (Bauman, 2007; Gee, 2003). Hiding Easter eggs in the digital environment can encourage self-guided orientation of virtual spaces. The Easter egg technique is not new or novel to video games. The 1979 Atari video game *Adventure* is thought to be the first video game to include an Easter egg as part of the game code and experience. In this quest-style game, the game developer, Warren Robinett, included a secret room that contained his signature "... created by Warren Robinett" (Robinett, 2006, pp. 712–713).

The Easter egg technique is a form of positive reinforcement. As a real-world example, recall when the automated secure drug dispensers were introduced into practice. These machines, really nothing more than secure vending machines, caused much anxiety for nurses who never used anything more automated than an IV pump, telephone, or call light in practice. During the training and early introduction phases of these machines, pharmacists and technicians were known to load spaces within the machine with bite-sized candy bars. This technique, while nothing more than a variation on providing an M&M to a child as positive reinforcement, was extremely popular and successful. Yet this Easter egg hunt, if you will, encouraged the use of new technology that transformed the clinical workplace by providing better pharmaceutical accountability and decreasing patient medication errors.

Encouraging self-orientation and providing guided orientation for novel teaching spaces is important because while most students are digital natives, some of your students may be digital immigrants (Prensky, 2001), that is to say they may be new to the digital world. Further, even if all of your students fit the mold of the digital native generation, some of these students may have other barriers that limit anecdotal or tacit knowledge of digital media. These barriers may be related to socio-economic status, culture, and availability of resources in students' homes or even hometowns. Without access to technology in and out of the classroom, the impact of developing technology can be negligible (Norris, Sullivan, Poirot, & Soloway, 2003).

Despite a boom in mobile device proliferation, the level of access to reliable Internet connectivity in many places in the United States and internationally remains unreliable and inadequate for many of the applications we hope to integrate into curricula. The point is that it is inappropriate to make assumptions about learners' experience with digital media and virtual spaces. While many contemporary educators see digital literacy as essential to academic success, we should not evaluate the ability to succeed globally based on students' past experience with digital technology. Given the opportunity, smart people will learn how to leverage digital technology to meet their goals. To do so they need adequate orientation, troubleshooting support, and a practice level or sandbox area to master necessary skills to function within the learning environment through ungraded practice.

THE ROLE OF INSTRUCTIONAL TECHNOLOGY AND DESIGN SUPPORT

Instructional Technology

Institutions use this term very broadly, generally as an all-encompassing term. In Chapter 2 we used the term *informational technology* and coupled it with the abbreviation IT. This said, defining "IT" as a stand-alone term is not helpful and likely is not possible. A Google search for the term *define IT* yields 138,000 results with the first result defining "IT" as a pronoun (www.dictionary.com). Farther down the Google findings, "IT" is defined in terms of informational technologies and just about everything pertaining to computers and the transfer of information from one source to another. The IT field encompasses a lot of content and means different things to different people. Cliché, but perhaps not too far from the truth, many have the perception that if something is plugged in or requires electricity to run, it falls under the domain of the IT department.

For the general purposes of this text we have defined IT or information technology as the acquisition, processing, storage, and use of information (in any format) by computers and telecommunications technology. From this perspective IT is more than hardware and software. Technology can be physical like a smartphone or it can be the application placed on the smartphone to leverage some sort of information. In reality, the IT system is more than the sum of its hard and soft parts.

Instructional Design

For the purposes of this text we have defined the term *instructional design* as the practice of implementing pedagogy using a systemic approach that is effective and efficient for teachers while being appealing to learners. ID is often used with online and new media sources, but can refer to any form of instruction or other learning experience. ID is an essential and often overlooked variable associated with the effective implementation of new media tools related to simulation and game-based learning. Very well-versed IT professionals who specialize in the movement, processing, and storage of information likely do not have specific training related to the design and implementation, integration, and evaluation of new and novel technology into new and existing curricula. Installing the software updates on a $100,000 mannikin-based simulator is one thing; knowing how to integrate the mannikin-based simulator into the curriculum to enhance and drive outcome is something entirely different. In this same vein, downloading the CliniSpace™ software, a virtual clinical training space, and configuring computer settings so this software will run effectively is an IT function. Working with teaching faculty and staff to effectively integrate CliniSpace™ into lesson plans to meet curriculum objectives requires ID expertise.

Just as there are professionals who specialize in IT, there are professionals who specialize in ID. The two types of expertise are not mutually exclusive. Today's successful instructional designers will generally have a high level of media and technology literacy. The most robust and efficient models for the development, integration, and support of game and simulation technology include a combination of content expertise, instructional design, and information technology.

Figure 4.1 provides a linear model or equation for successful integration of games and simulation into any curriculum. If you are using a linear model it is important to begin with content and objectives and progress toward the instructional design process, and finally figure out the technical aspects of integrations. While this model is simple, it does provide a starting place for process integration and accounts for the minimum assets required to plan, deploy, and evaluate game-based learning (Figure 4.1).

Figure 4.2 represents a more collaborative model for technology integration success. In this model the content expertise, instructional design, and information technology facets are represented in a Venn diagram. The area of the diagram where content expertise, instructional design, and informational technology overlap represents the "sweet spot" for success. The collaborative approach has several advantages. Digital learning spaces are dynamic. Integrating simulation and game-based learning requires more forethought and ongoing support than integrating a new textbook into a syllabus or curriculum. Moving forward without an inclusive conversation that includes content experts (faculty), instructional designers, and information technologists often yields

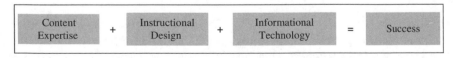

FIGURE 4.1
Linear model for technology integration success

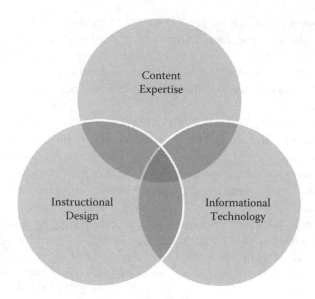

FIGURE 4.2
Collaborative model for technology integration success

unforeseen challenges. When all of these elements are seen as valuable parts of the integration process from the onset, educators can address pedagogy, design, hardware, and software variables efficiently to support best practice and outcome throughout the planning, implementation, and evaluation process. A collaborative process can mitigate misunderstanding and support realistic expectations related to all elements of the educational intervention (Figure 4.2).

Getting Started: Repurposing Existing Technology and Exploring New Technology

Other chapters of this book will provide examples of repurposing different types of software and commercial video games to promote and achieve objectives situated within the context of nursing and other types of clinical and health sciences education. Chapter 2 provided an example of using presentation software to facilitate leaning objectives among education students. Chapter 3 discussed how Sid Meier's game, *Civilization* has been used to teach history among primary education students. Chapter 8 will provide a theoretical case study of how a game like *Starcraft 2* can be used to promote nontechnical skills like critical decision making.

While the authors of this textbook support the innovative repurposing of all sorts of multimedia software including commercial video games for learning, we would not suggest that readers rush out to buy all of the latest game titles and evaluate them for merit within the context of their course and curriculum. Those institutions that are already using simulation as an integral part of their curriculum can repurpose the software used to run their mannikin-based simulators for various lessons related to basic and applied physiology and pharmacology.

The METI/CAE Müse and HPS (Human Patient Simulator) software models physiology and allows the operator to modify physiologic parameters to provide a representative physiologic response to various drugs. Even novice operators are able to use this software to discuss the well-known, essential formula and concept of cardiac output. Cardiac output is a function of heart rate multiplied by stroke volume (HR × SV = Cardiac Output). As heart rate increases, stroke volume decreases. In general, when stroke volume increases, heart rate decreases. This concept can be difficult to teach, but is essential to many facets of applied cardio-respiratory physiology. Cardiac output is affected by any number of disease processes, related physiological states, and medications.

The Müse and HPS software allows the instructor to manipulate physiology in response to pathology and related treatment interventions and display them on a patient monitor in real time or through the magic of technology in an accelerated manner. Because the physiology and display are virtual, the location of the lesson becomes irrelevant. Because the patient data can be decoupled from the mannikin and used in an entirely virtual sense, students can engage many "if then" scenarios and simply reset the patient as needed with the click of a mouse (Figure 4.3 and Figure 4.4).

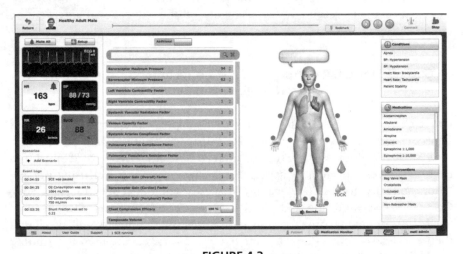

FIGURE 4.3

Screen capture of METI/CAE Müse software in the advanced cardiac parameters operator control screen

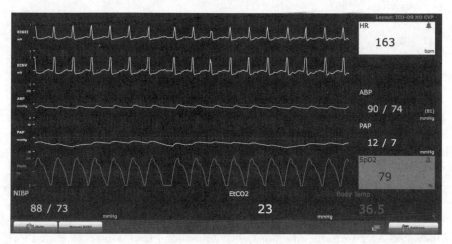

FIGURE 4.4
Screen capture of METI/CAE TouchPro virtual monitor

Repurposing a mannikin-based simulator in this manner incorporates facets of the "good game." Students are encouraged to explore, to leave no stone unturned, and experiment—with no dangerous consequences for patients. This sort of repurposing brings an entirely new level of engagement to case-based learning. Instructors become facilitators of knowledge acquisition, rather than the tellers of facts. The phrase, ". . . why don't you rethink that" morphs into ". . . let's see what happens if we do that." Because this example of repurposing decouples the Müse and HPS software from the mannikin, it is possible to incorporate the simulation in a virtual context into the general classroom, as a part of real-time distance learning, and during study groups and small group discussions taking place outside of the confines of the physical simulation laboratory.

One frequently asked question related to games and health sciences education is, "Where do I actually find games that I can play now and immediately integrate into my curriculum?" This textbook provides an appendix of available ready-to-go games. Readers should take care to play and evaluate each game for its relevance to course content and objectives.

The ongoing Games and Simulation for Healthcare online library and database (http://healthcaregames.wisc.edu/) hosted by the Ebling Health Sciences Library at the University of Wisconsin aims to provide a portal and network to meet the needs of clinicians, researchers, and educators in the healthcare community who want to integrate games and simulation into their scholarship and patient care strategy. This database is searchable and includes many ready-to-use games. Several additional resources can be found in Table 4.1.

TABLE 4.1
Healthcare Games

Health Games Research	http://healthgamesresearch.org/
healthGAMERS	www.healthgamers.com/
Games for Health	www.gamesforhealth.org/
Virtual Anesthesia Machine and Simulation Portfolio—University of Florida	http://vam.anest.ufl.edu/

Establishing a Continuum of Introduction and Integration of Game-Based Learning Into Your Curriculum

Once you have introduced games and simulations into your course or more broadly across a curriculum, it is worthwhile and necessary to maintain current technology and introduce new technology. There is often an up-front cost—monetary and human resources—to introducing simulation and game-based learning into and across curricula. Once this infrastructure is in place, neglecting the content, pedagogy, or delivery mechanism can be costly. The analogy is akin to paying a company to build a multifaceted website to show-case a school or business, but spending little or no effort in developing new and current content. Once the user experience gets stale, there is little reason to visit the website. Or worse yet, the website is not maintained from an infrastructure perspective and it becomes unreliable and unusable.

We discussed repurposing in the previous section of this chapter. Repurposing is an efficient way to leverage current technology in ways that develop new content for your curriculum. Leveraging what you have first before moving on to new technology helps teachers and administrators make decisions about the selection and integration of future technology that supports not only game-based learning, but the overall objectives of the curriculum. The "build it and they will come" method of technology is naïve and expensive. A combination of student, school, and curriculum objectives and future employer expectations should drive the introduction, integration, and analysis of games and simulations into and throughout the curriculum.

New products and multimedia technology, once selected, should be tested and evaluated by teaching faculty and staff prior to introduction to the student population. Faculty should be prepared to modify and improve the way any given game or simulation is being used over time. Many experienced leaders in the game and simulation industry are constantly refining and introducing facets to existing games and simulations. The key here is not to try out new games or refined experiences without rehearsal on "live" students. In fact, it is helpful to let students know when they are the first group or early group of students walking through a new virtual environment or game experience. This abates unrealistic student expectations and provides you with the opportunity to glean important feedback about how the designed experience has played with learners.

Once a program has established a reputation for innovation and leadership related to novel learning pedagogy, current and future students, as well as peer institutions, will expect you to maintain your reputation. Those who are interested in the concept of teaching and learning in new and novel ways must become aware that it is no longer appropriate to assume schools will drive student expectations. The best and brightest students will drive curricula and have expectations about how that curriculum should be delivered.

Employers, including hospitals, are often more nimble in the acquisition and leveraging of new technology. Further, employers are going to influence educational delivery because they drive practice expectations. Meeting entry-to-practice expectations means that schools will need to be accepting of multimedia learning experiences because students' future employers are already integrating novel approaches to not only clinical education, but also patient education. Introducing game-based learning and leveraging innovative technology including mobile technology and applications is becoming a necessity in terms of professional media literacy. Media literacy in the context of game-based applications is becoming an expectation for professional practice.

SUMMARY

This chapter has discussed essential elements needed to prepare faculty and students for game-based pedagogies. The chapter began by addressing the importance of faculty engagement and buy-in when embracing new and novel technology such as simulation and game-based learning. This section discussed the importance of leveraging existing experts and provided strategies for developing expertise among less initiated faculty. The chapter also emphasized the importance of learner readiness. Both faculty and students come to learning environments with previous experience that will drive their expectations. The chapter introduced the readers to the concepts of the digital native and digital immigrant (Prensky 2001, 2010) and suggested that students are more likely to be digital natives, while faculty are more likely to be digital immigrants. However, the chapter emphasized that there can be a breadth of digital literacy among both students and faculty.

The discussion later moved to stress the importance of both technology and design support. Information technology and instructional design are not the same thing, albeit the two areas of expertise are not mutually exclusive. The successful approaches to the integration of simulation and game-based pedagogy and activities into curricula requires a combination of three areas of expertise: content, instructional design, and informational technology. Both a linear and collaborative model to the integration of these facets was discussed, with a preference for the collaborative approach.

The chapter provided a discussion about getting started and repurposing existing technology in ways that support game-based learning. To this end, several resources and databases were discussed to provide the reader with additional capital. In addition, a games resource appendix for this text provides a list of many ready-to-go games that can be incorporated into curricula. Also, this chapter included an example of how to repurpose existing mannikin-based software as a multimedia tool to support additional learning experiences for students. Other examples of repurposing existing software and commercial video games are seeded throughout the text.

Finally, this chapter suggests that successful programs will come to offer a continuum of game-based learning experiences throughout their curriculum. As technology continues to advance, learners will come to programs with expectations of how content will be delivered and mastered. Community stakeholders, specifically the future employers of your students, will also expect that students enter the workforce with a certain level of digital literacy. The chapter argues that game-based learning provides an avenue to meet this expectation. Faculty who gain a reputation for innovative and effective teaching will be sought after by students and other faculty hoping to find new ways, perhaps more effective ways, to engage students. In turn, schools and colleges who support simulation and game-based learning through IT infrastructure and ID support, as well as a culture of acceptance, will assume leadership roles among their peer institutions and be better positioned to attract the best and brightest students and faculty.

REFERENCES

Aleckson, J., & Ralston-Berg, P. (2011). *Micro-collaboration between eLearning designers and instructor experts.* Madison, WI: Atwood Publishing.

Baranowski, T., Buday, R., Thompson, D. I., & Baranowski, J. (2008). Playing for real: Video games and stories for health-related behavior change. *American Journal of Preventative Medicine, 34*(1), 74–82.

Bauman, E. (2007). *High fidelity simulation in healthcare.* PhD dissertation, The University of Wisconsin—Madison, United States. Dissertations & Theses @ CIC Institutions database. (Publication no. AAT 3294196 ISBN: 9780549383109 ProQuest document ID: 1453230861)

Bauman, E. (2010). Virtual reality and game-based clinical education. In K. B. Gaberson & M. H. Oermann (Eds.) *Clinical teaching strategies in nursing education* (3rd ed.) New York, Springer: Publishing Company.

Benner, P. (1984). From novice to expert: Excellence and power in clinical nursing practice. Menlo Park, CA: Addison-Wesley.

Cooper, J. B., & Taqueti, V. R. (2004). A brief history of the development of mannequin simulators for clinical education and training. *Quality and Safety in Health Care, 13*(Suppl. 1), i11–i18.

Gee, J. P. (2003). *What video games have to teach us about learning literacy.* New York: Palgrave MacMillian.

Gee, J. P. (2004). Learning by design: Games for as learning machines. *Interactive Educational Multimedia*, 8(April), 15–23.

Gisondi, M. A., Smith-Coggins, R., Harter, P. M., Soltysik, R. C., & Yarnold, P. R. (2004) Assessment of resident professionalism using high-fidelity simulation of ethical dilemmas. *Academic Emergency Medicine*, *11*, 931–937.

Greenfield, P. M. (2010). Video games revisited. In R. Van Eck (Ed.), *Gaming and cognition: Theories and practice from the learning sciences*. Hershey, PA: IGI Global.

Grenvik, A., & Schaefer, J. (2004). From resusci-anne to sim-man: The evolution of simulators in medicine. *Critical Care Medicine*, *32*(Suppl. 2), S56–S57.

Hayes, E. (2005). Women, video gaming and learning: Beyond stereotypes. *TechTrends*, *49*(5), 23–28.

Kron, F. W., Gjerde, C. L., Sen, A., & Fetters, M. D. (2010). Medical student attitudes toward video games and new media technologies in medical education. *BMJ Medical Education*, *10*(1), 50–60.

Lenhart, A, Jones, S., & Mcgill, A. J. (2008). *Adults and video games*. Washing D.C.: Pew Internet and American Life Project.

Lieberman, D. A. (2009). Designing serious games for health in informal and formal settings. In U. Ritterfeld, M. Cody & P. Vorderer (Eds). *Serious games: mechanisms and effects*. New York: Routledge.

Norris, C., Sullivan, T., Poirot, J., & Soloway, E. (2003). No access, no use, no impact: Snapshot surveys of educational technology in K-12. *Journal of Research on Technology in Education*, 6(21), 15–27.

Prensky, M. (2001). Digital natives, digital immigrants part 1. *On the Horizon*, 9(5), 2–6.

Prensky, M. (2010). *Teaching digital natives: Partnering for real learning*. Corwin Press.

Robinett, W. (2006). Adventure as a Video Game: Adventure for the Atari 2600. In Salen, K., & Zimmerman, E., (Eds.), *The game design reader: A rules of play anthology*. Cambridge, MA: MIT Press.

Schön, D. A. (1983). The reflective practitioner: How professionals think in action. New York: Basic Books.

Shaffer, D. W., Squire, K. D., Halverson, R., & Gee, J. P. (2005). Video games and the future of learning. *Phi Delta Kappan*, *87*(2), 104–111.

Squire, K. (2003). Video games in education. *International Journal of Intelligent Games & Simulation*, *2*(1), 49–62.

Squire, K. (2006). From content to context: Videogames as designed experience. *Educational Researcher*, *35*(8), 19–29.

Telner, D., Bujas-Bobanovic, M., Chan, D., Chester, B., Marlow Meuser, B. et al. (2010). Game-based versus traditional case-based learning: comparing effectiveness in stroke continuing medical education. *Canadian Family Physician*, *59*(9), e345–e351.

Thiagarajan, S. (1992). Using games for debriefing. *Simulation and Gaming*, *23*, 161–173.

Tyczkowski, B., Bauman, E., Gallagher-Lepak, S., Vandenhouten, C., & Resop Reilly, J. (In Press). An interface design evaluation of courses in a nursing program using an e-learning framework: A case study. In Khan, B. (Ed.), *User interface design for virtual environments: Challenges and advances*. Washington, DC: McWeadon Press.

Williams, D., Martins, N., Conslavo, M., & Ivory, J. D. (2009). The virtual census: representations of gender, race and age in video games. *New Media & Society, 11*(15), 815–834.
Williams, D., Yee, N., & Caplan, S. E. (2008). Who plays, how much, and why? Debunking the stereotypical gamer profile. *Journal of Computer-Mediated Communication, 13*(4), 993–1018.

5

Using Virtual and Game-Based Learning to Prepare for Actual Practice

ERIC B. BAUMAN AND MOSES WOLFENSTEIN

OVERVIEW

*T*his chapter will discuss how educators can use virtual learning spaces and game-based learning to prepare students for actual practice settings and challenge readers to think about what counts as a learning space and clinical encounter. We will define and discuss the terms *environmental* and *psychological fidelity*. We also examine the important role that environmental and psychological fidelity plays in the context of game and simulation-based education and the relationship between the two, emphasizing the importance of fidelity and learners' ability to suspend their disbelief.

We also explore and emphasize the importance that context plays within created environments that are situated to actual clinical practice. Content is discussed as it relates to consistency with actual clinical environments and as a function of maintaining consistent educational experiences across the curriculum. Further this chapter presents game-based learning applications and digital platforms such as virtual reality as collaborative, synergistic tools for clinical education and preparedness.

Finally, this chapter discusses the role of game-based learning and simulation in the context of primary nursing, clinical education, and continuing education, as well as a mechanism for clinical threat assessment and patient

The authors acknowledge and thank Gerald Stapleton, Director of Distance Education at the University of Illinois, Chicago College of Medicine for providing the digital/virtual world images for this chapter.

safety. We provide theoretical and existing case studies to emphasize how educators integrate simulation and game-based learning. We discuss how they might be used in existing curricula and how these tools can transform opportunities for increased patient safety.

LEARNING SPACES

Nursing programs exist in a variety of different institutions. Many nurses still practicing today received their initial nurse's training in traditional 3-year diploma programs that were associated with or existed as part of a hospital. While these programs have been phased out, primary nursing education continues to exist in 2-year Associate degree programs often associated with technical or community colleges and at 4-year baccalaureate nursing programs offered at many colleges and universities. Master's-level and doctorate-level degree programs are now common in nursing. Many view graduate training as a normal progression for students entering the field including practicing nurses who wish to advance or redirect their role and scope of practice.

Distance and distributive education models are not new to nursing from either the primary/pre-licensure or continuing education perspective (Armstrong, Gessner, & Skott Cooper, 2000). However, what is new to nursing education is the role that innovative technology plays in the way that content is delivered and distributed. New and emerging technology directly impacts how educators facilitate distance education and how it might affect future online learning. Online or *e-Learning* (discussed in more detail in Chapter 6) is reframing student and faculty expectations for academic achievement. Historically, students could complete associate and baccalaureate didactic nursing credits though correspondence courses. Now e-Learning and online *Learning Management Systems* are transforming both the undergraduate and higher education landscapes. The transformation is forcing educators to rethink not only what counts for academic achievement, but also what counts for classroom and clinical learning experiences.

Mannikin-Based Laboratories

Many nursing schools, medical schools, and other allied health sciences programs now embrace and integrate mannikin-based simulation into their curricula (Gaba, 2004; Gore, Van Gele, Ravert & Mabire, in press). Some clinical disciplines including anesthesia now require simulation-based continuing education experiences to maintain clinical certifications (Boulet & Murray, 2010; Gallagher & Tan, 2010). Nursing laboratories have long been accepted and common learning spaces. Traditional nursing laboratories represent spaces where educators continue to use *low-fidelity* or static mannikins and even *partial task trainers* to teach students psychomotor skills associated with nursing. However, the contemporary mannikin-based high-fidelity simulation laboratories are *created spaces*. They are used to facilitate *designed experiences* that are authentically situated to target nursing and other clinical disciplines. The contemporary simulation laboratory is more akin to the immersive environment portrayed on the holodeck found in the science fiction franchise *Star Trek*. The *Star Trek* holodeck provides an embodied, immersive environment indistinguishable from the real world. The perfect simulation lab would provide an experience like the holodeck. It would be indistinguishable from reality (Bauman, 2007; Gaba 2004).

While the fixed physical space of the contemporary simulation laboratory is quickly becoming a standard of educational practice for clinical education, it is still a relatively new method of instruction. Ten years ago, at best the number of schools using high-fidelity mannikin-based simulation was scant. Five years ago, more innovative and technically progressive schools began integrating mannikin-based simulation into their curricula in limited capacities. The number of nursing schools and other health sciences schools now building high-fidelity simulation laboratories is exploding.

Game-Based and Virtual Reality Learning Spaces

Game-based learning and virtual-reality learning experiences are the new novel technology presenting itself to nursing and other forms of clinical education. As previously discussed and emphasized throughout this text, digital environments presented as either stand-alone games or as part of virtual worlds address the challenges of location and time related to clinical education. Mannikin-based simulation occurring in situ or within contemporary simulation laboratories provides a milieu of consistency not available in actual clinical environments (Bauman, 2007; Friedrich, 2002; Gordon, Oriol, & Cooper, 2004; Lane, Slavin, & Ziv, 2001; Shapiro & Simmons, 2002; Ziv, Wolpe, Small & Glick, 2003). That said, fixed space and in situ simulations only provide educational experiences to learners that are fixed in terms of time and location. Game-based experiences and those experiences occurring in virtual worlds reframe the time and location paradigm.

Augmented Reality

Augmented reality supplements the *real world*. Actual objects existing in the *real world* appear to coexist with virtual objects, computer-generated images that are representations of actual objects. Augmented reality supplements reality rather than providing an independent immersive virtual environment. In a virtual environment, as in a game-based environment, individuals are entirely immersed. In other words, they are not interacting in the real world around them. When using *augmented reality*, individuals or learners remain in and see the *real world*, with virtual objects superimposed upon or blended within the real world (Azuma, 1997). According to Azuma, Baillot, Behringer, Feiner, Julier, and MacIntrye (2001), augmented reality systems are defined by the following three properties:

- A combination of real and virtual objects coexisting in a real environment.
- The environment is interactive and exists in real time.
- Real and virtual objects register or align with each other.

Augmented reality adds facets of the real world that are not always available at a given time or place, particularly in educational settings. Augmented reality can be used to supplement fixed learning settings like mannikin-based or in situ simulations to drive fidelity and provide cues or cognitive aids for learners. Further, augmented reality has the potential to transcend initial and continuing education learning experiences and advance actual clinical practice. Advances in virtual and augmented reality are able to create realistic imitations of surgical procedures (Kneebone, Scott, Darzi, & Horrocks, 2004, p. 38). Further, *augmented reality* can provide visual cues in preparation for and during surgical and other invasive procedures. These cues may represent virtual anatomical models specific to actual patients and can provide heads-up displays of cognitive aides during procedures so that clinicians need not look away from a surgical field to access case-related information (Azuma, 1997).

WHAT COUNTS: SIMULATION, GAME-BASED LEARNING AND CLINICAL HOURS

Simulation as Clinical Education

Simulation activities occurring in a laboratory or in situ feel more like clinical encounters than didactic modalities of education like lecture and small group discussion. Simulation-based experiences, whether they exist in fixed spaces (the laboratory or in situ) or in virtual spaces (online or within a digital game space), can be designed to have clinical value and utility. Simulations can be designed and implemented across curricula to provide just-in-time consistent clinical experiences to complement didactic content. They can be customized, designed, and individualized to fill gaps in students' real-world clinical experiences. The point is that simulation-based education is clinical education. Some may argue that it is difficult to evaluate and guarantee the quality of clinical simulations existing in actual or virtual spaces. However, the quality and constancy dilemma also exists with traditional real-world clinical experiences. Yet simulation guarantees that all students have access to the same clinical cases, cases that are seen as essential experiences for entry to practice. This type of consistency cannot be guaranteed during actual supervised clinical rotations.

Nursing schools and other clinical training centers, including emergency medical services (EMS) programs, are debating the number of simulation hours that translate to or can be counted as supervised clinical hours. Nursing and other clinical sciences require students to complete supervised clinical hours. The number of hours varies based on the level (undergraduate versus graduate) and type (nursing, EMS, medical) education.

The percentage or number of hours in which actual real-world clinical hours may be substituted with simulation-based experiences is inconsistent. (Gore et al., in press). For example, international regulatory bodies and the state Boards of Nursing for differing states throughout the United States have come to different conclusions as to the percent or number of simulation-based hours that can count toward students' clinical experience. Many Boards of Nursing in the United States and international regulatory bodies contain no rules or opinions related to simulation-based instruction in their administrative code or guidelines (Hayden, 2010). In Utah, the State Board of Nursing allows for a maximum of 25% of clinical hours obtained in nursing skills laboratories or through simulation or virtual excursions (Utah Nurse Practice Act, 2012). In the United Kingdom up to 300 h of the 2,300 h practice component of pre-registration nursing training (in a three year program) can take place in a simulated practice environment (Nursing & Midwifery Council, 2007).

The same conundrum also exists in EMS training. For example, in Wisconsin students enrolled in EMS training, including paramedic-level training, can count simulation-based training as clinical experience. In Wisconsin, the state paramedic curriculum has moved away from a stated hours-based clinical curriculum to a competency-based curriculum. Further, educators may use simulation to demonstrate competency and count it for a significant amount of explicitly stated clinical contacts. For example "... up to one-half of the listed competency requirement may be obtained through scenario-based, high-fidelity simulation-based experiences" (Wisconsin Department of Health Services, WMS Section, 2011). At first glance this sort of simulation for clinical hour substitution may seem entirely irrational. However, the nature of paramedic clinical encounters are inconsistent. Students may spend eight or more hours in an emergency department or assigned to clinical mentors in the field without any actual clinical encounters taking place. In other instances, students only encounter clinical experiences of limited complexity. Using simulations to ensure consistent clinical encounters better prepares students for actual practice environments when the alternative is considered; no hands-on clinical encounter, virtual or otherwise. *Designed experiences* existing in *created environments* certainly offer more complexity, utility, and value than no encounter at all.

Accreditation and Certification

Various educationally focused professional societies are establishing certification and accreditation guidelines for aspects of simulation-based activities. Accreditation refers to an institution's simulation program and facilities. The

Society for Simulation in Healthcare (SSH) and the International Nursing Association of Clinical Leaning and Simulation (INACSL) established guidelines and categories for program accreditation including teaching/education, research, assessment, and systems integration (Faragher, Boese, Decker, & Sando, 2011; Society for Simulation in Healthcare, Council for Accreditation of Healthcare Simulation Programs, 2012).

In the context of this discussion, "certification" refers to the instructor. Similarly, "instructor" refers to those facilitating learning activities using simulation as a method of instruction, whether the instruction is taking place in a fixed laboratory or in a virtual or game-based environment. The SSH is developing a simulation instructor certification process. State Boards of Nursing and accrediting agencies in the United States provide standards that define the requirements for nursing instructors. In general, nursing instructors must earn and possess a master's degree in nursing prior to teaching undergraduate or pre-licensure nursing courses. While some exceptions exist, a master's degree in nursing generally defines the teaching requirement for instructors in undergraduate nursing programs. Certification in the method of instruction, in this case, simulation, represents a specialty teaching credential. Certification in this case will likely represent a teaching credential that moves beyond state requirements and provides evidence of professional expertise.

Instructor certification is not a new concept in the realm of clinical education. The American Heart Association (AHA) requires those teaching AHA courses, including but not limited to Basic Life Support, Advanced Cardiac Life Support, and Pediatric Advanced Life Support be recognized AHA instructors who have demonstrated content and teaching expertise specific to the courses they teach. However, students enrolled in these courses are earning a "branded" specialty credential or designation that indicates that they have successfully completed a prescribed AHA course. Providing a simulation instructor with certification focuses less on content and more on pedagogy and demonstrated ability, proficiency, and expertise within the domain of simulation-based education.

RETHINKING LEARNING SPACES: FIDELITY, SUSPENSION OF DISBELIEF, AND THEATRICS

Fidelity: Environmental and Psychological

Fidelity in the context of simulation is often discussed from two perspectives, *environmental fidelity* and *psychological fidelity*. For the purposes of this textbook we have defined *environmental fidelity* as it relates to the physical surroundings, representation, and characteristics in which a simulation or game takes place (Bauman, 2007; Dieckmann, Gaba, & Rall, 2007; Gaba, 2004).

Gaba (2004) further discusses the role of realistic environmental immersion (environmental fidelity) as it relates to *suspension of disbelief*. Those environments that accurately represent practice or work environments are said to have high environmental fidelity. Gaba (2004) uses the fictional *Star Trek* holodeck as an example of a *created space* where immersion, or environmental fidelity is so accurate or complete that participants are unable to distinguish between the simulated environment and real life.

Psychological fidelity relates to an individual's ability to suspend disbelief in reality and become immersed in the situation (Bauman, 2007; Gee, 2003). In many cases increasing *environmental fidelity* will drive *psychological fidelity*. Issenberg and Scalese (2008) discuss *psychological fidelity* in the context of simulation-based training as "... the degree to which the trainee perceives the simulation to be a believable surrogate for the trained tasks (behavior). This can be maximized by developing simulation scenarios that mimic the task demands of the real process" (pp. 33–34).

Suspension of Disbelief

Suspension of disbelief is the product of adequate environmental and psychological fidelity. "... Experience shows that participants in immersive simulations easily suspend disbelief and speak and act much as they do in their real jobs" (Gaba, 2004, p. i2). In other words the *environmental fidelity* situates or drives *psychological fidelity*, which in turn encourages *suspension of disbelief* (Bauman, 2007; Flanagan, Nestel, & Joseph, 2004; Halamek et al., 2000; Seropian, 2003). Dieckmann et al. (2007) also discuss the phenomenal mode of simulation. The phenomenal mode of simulation relates to learners' emotions, beliefs, and cognitive states that take place during simulation. The *suspension of disbelief* encompasses or relates to the learner's or student's state of mind, such that the student may not be cognizant of facilitators and instructors. Figure 5.1 provides a diagram that illustrates variables that lead to suspension of disbelief. The cone represents the overall educational experience as perceived by the learner, and the spheres represent the perceptions of environmental and psychological fidelity.

Theatrics

One of the common mistakes that many novices to simulation make is that they assume *high-fidelity* is required to achieve suspension of disbelief. This is not the case. The ability to situate learning experiences and achieve suspension of disbelief depends on tasks, lessons, and objectives. To this point *theatrics* are as important, perhaps even more important to achieving the *suspension of disbelief* among students than the level of available fidelity. In general,

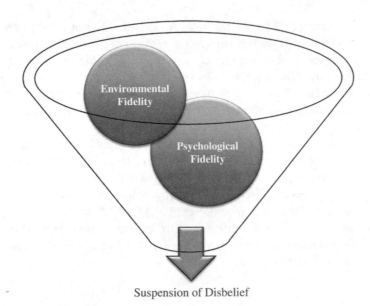

Suspension of Disbelief

FIGURE 5.1

Process illustration for Suspension of Disbelief (Images provided by Gerald Stapleton, University of Illinois at Chicago, 2012)

"high fidelity" refers to simulators or environments that are model driven (Maran & Glavin 2003). High fidelity simulators and environments are interactive and responsive; they will respond to the actions or inactions of learners.

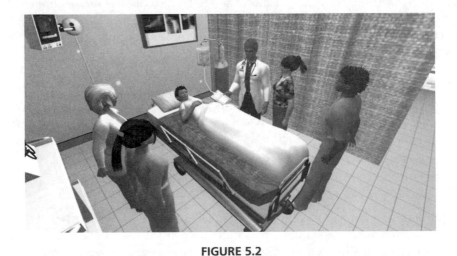

FIGURE 5.2

Clinicians in a virtual world environment with appropriate avatar characteristics and dress attire (Images provided by Gerald Stapleton, University of Illinois at Chicago, 2012)

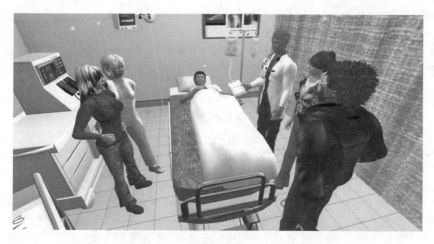

FIGURE 5.3

Clinicians in a virtual world environment with appropriate avatar characteristics and inappropriate dress attire. Note that the two avatars in the foreground on the left and right are dressed in inappropriate clinical attire. However, this sort of attire might be acceptable for in-world characters playing the role of patient, family member, or friend. (Images provided by Gerald Stapleton, University of Illinois at Chicago, 2012)

High-fidelity simulators and environments provide learners with experiences that move beyond task training. Low-fidelity simulators allow students to explore basic-level, unidimensional skills while high-fidelity simulators and

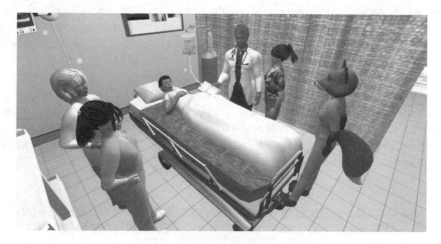

FIGURE 5.4

Clinicians in a virtual world environment in appropriate dress attire and one avatar with inappropriate physical characteristics. Note the shocked look on the patient's face. (Images provided by Gerald Stapleton, University of Illinois at Chicago, 2012)

environments encourage students to explore complex multidimensional skills. Complex skills include communication and behavioral skills associated with teamwork and leadership, while providing patient care (Bauman, 2007). High-fidelity simulators provide ongoing and immediate feedback as learning experiences progress (Lane et al., 2001).

It is important to realize created environments are inherently theatrical. Not every piece of equipment in a fixed-space simulation laboratory has to be a functional piece of medical equipment. For example, is it necessary to have a real $50,000 defibrillator bedside in the simulation laboratory or will a Hollywood-style theatrical prop work just as well (Dieckmann et al., 2007)? The answer depends on what the objective of the lesson is. If the objective is to orient students to the actual defibrillator they will use in clinical practice in the near future, the relevance of the defibrillator becomes much more important than if the objective of the lesson is to situate learners to a working emergency department or intensive care unit.

The same paradigm exists in virtual environments. Not every object visible in a virtual environment has to be "clickable" or interactive in order to set the stage for an authentic encounter that encourages suspension of disbelief among learners. The role that theatrics plays in simulation and game-based learning is illustrated by comparing a well-executed play to a multi-million dollar bad movie. Money spent on special effects cannot substitute for the plot, quality of acting, and story line. Many people have walked out of movie theaters in spite of the theatrics, but have been captivated and on the edge of their seats during traditional theatrical productions. High fidelity alone does not drive learner experience. The appropriate and well-executed use of a prop or environment may in fact provide a more cost-effective and better experience than an actual piece of equipment or a lesson provided in an actual clinical environment. Use theatrics to convince learners that their environment is authentic, but understand that the created environment will not be and need not be completely authentic. Further, beginning students may find authentic environments that provide all the variables of actual practice very distracting. The stage and associated theatrics of the lesson plan should map back to lesson objectives. Complicating teaching environments designed for novice learners with multiple variables yields ineffective learning opportunities and frustrated students.

ACCESS TO VIRTUAL ENVIRONMENTS: SAFETY, ACCULTURATION, CONSISTENCY, BEST PRACTICES, AND MAINTENANCE

We must continually evaluate and monitor the virtual environment where learning takes place. Fixed-space classrooms are often static and come with a well-understood set of rules and social mores. Learners must see and interpret virtual environments as safe learning spaces from various perspectives.

Further, because these spaces often exist when instructional staff are not present, the environment should be engineered to provide consistency whether direct clinical supervision is or is not present. Assurances that curricula objectives and best practices are promoted whenever the environment is accessible requires continual assessment, evaluation, and a commitment to ongoing quality improvement.

Safety

When we address the concept of safety broadly in the context of higher education, most people think about physical safety of students on campus. From the healthcare perspective, safety is most often thought about in terms of patient safety as it relates to quality assurance. However, from an educational perspective, safety also relates to the emotional well-being of the learner (Erickson, Fox, & Stewart, 2010; Gamage, Tretiakov, & Crump, 2011). Many campuses in K – 12 and increasingly in higher education now address emotional safety in terms of bullying behavior and inappropriate discriminatory behavior that affects students' emotional or psychological well-being. It is equally important to be cognizant of emotional and psychological safety when students are engaged in learning activities that are or can become highly charged, or include some sort of deception in order to facilitate experiences that situate course objectives (Bauman, 2007; Thiagarajan, 1992). Virtual environments offer a sense of co-presence, or sense of togetherness. It is very important that educators and administrators account for emotional safety in digital social spaces used for academic purposes because educators have both an implicit and explicit responsibility for student safety. Put simply, teachers have an obligation to promote safety in educational spaces. Without significant forethought, virtual campuses may lack the same sort of obvious control and consequence that exist on a real-world campus, particularly when teachers and faculty are not always present alongside learners in digital environments.

As discussed throughout this text, simulation and game-based learning is inherently experiential. Experiential learning activities occur through self-guided and facilitated debriefing. While many instructors see debriefing as part of the educational process, it must also provide the opportunity for faculty to check in with students to assess students' emotional status at the conclusion of simulation or game sessions. When conducting simulation and game-based research associated with human subject experimentation, debriefings should undo any deception and counter any actual negative or perceived negative consequences (Bauman, 2007; Stewart, 1992).

Further, plans submitted to institutional review boards must provide a clear mechanism to address the emotional and physical safety of students/subjects participating in any form of research. We argue that educational interventions should follow basic principles associated with human subject best practices. Immersive educational encounters are more emotionally engaging than static activities, particularly during encounters that deal with emotionally charged events like death and dying, medication errors, and social mores (Leighton & Dubas, 2009; Sperlazza & Cangelosi, 2009; Thiagarajan, 1992). This may be as simple as having a referral plan in place so that educators can easily refer students to the appropriate campus student services program.

For example, take into consideration the following scenario. A participant in a continuing education course on the topic of advanced cardiac life support leaves a simulation session in tears and declines to participate in the rest of the course despite potential negative professional consequences. The simulation session the nurse was participating in was not a high-stakes examination, but rather a learning station that teaches participants objectives related to sudden cardiac arrest. At the time of this incident the emotional response of the student seemed entirely out of context. However, follow-up with the student by the nursing supervisor and the course medical director yield that the student has himself suffered sudden cardiac arrest with a successful resuscitation and the mere content of the lesson triggered a post-traumatic stress response.

In another example, a nursing student becomes very defensive and tearful over feedback provided about the administration of a medication in a game-based learning environment. She is argumentative and leaves the session complaining how inappropriate the instructor/facilitator was and says she is done with "stupid" pretend clinical sessions. Further investigation of the situation finds that in an actual supervised clinical this student witnessed a medication error that led to a negative patient outcome. The current learning activity evoked a strong emotional response.

As teachers, faculty, and administrators, we are rarely aware of the lived experiences of our students. Yet past experience will shape current and future experiences. As nurses and clinicians we have ethical and moral responsibilities to our patients. As teachers we have ethical and moral responsibilities to our students. Virtual environments present some very real challenges to student emotional safety and well-being because virtual and game-based environments are dynamic and persistent. That is, once a participant or learner is immersed in a virtual environment, we as instructors loose some control over the dynamics of the situation.

Acculturation

Virtual learning spaces provide opportunities to acculturate nursing students for the expectations and social mores associated with professional nursing. These environments provide students with the opportunity to actually be a nurse in ways not available to students in real-world clinical encounters. In the real world, nursing students can play only one role. In essence, they cannot be the registered nurses of record. They are identified by name tag and often uniform as a student nurse. Designed clinical learning activities taking place in virtual environments provide nursing students with important professional cues related to the conduct associated with the profession that they are seeking to join. The game narrative drives learning through designed and targeted learning activities. Because teachers and instructional designers are privy to the narrative theme and lesson objectives unfolding during simulation and game-based learning activities, they can guide students through situated contexts of practice whether these practice elements are task or behavioral in nature (Bauman, 2010; Games & Bauman, 2011; Gee, 2003).

As previously discussed, virtual and game-based learning environments are dynamic and often malleable. By malleable we mean that those immersed in the environment can contribute to the environment. The easiest way that participants contribute to their environments is through appearance. Many video games and virtual worlds have extensive avatar modeling capabilities. Players often spend hours getting their look just right. Some will choose to model their avatar after their real-world appearance, many will not. In the game world, appearance moves beyond clothing and accessory selection and crosses gender and ethnic boundaries. Player appearance can and does cross species boundaries in some game worlds. The potential for avatar flexibility and malleability in virtual worlds coupled with anonymity can lead to contextually inappropriate behavior, particularly in teaching spaces designed to acculturate students to professional practice (Bauman, 2010).

Institutions already provide guidelines or rules of conduct for various learning spaces. The dress code for the classroom is different than the dress code for clinical sites. Many schools and institutions require the same dress code for clinical encounters taking place in fixed-simulation laboratories as they do for actual clinical settings existing in hospitals, clinics, and the community. Given this practice, administrators may find it helpful to institute the same appearance policy for students engaging in clinical encounters and professional roles in the virtual world. The term "appearance policy" is deliberately chosen. Many immersive digital environments allow players to customize their *avatars*. When using existing environments such as *Second Life*, the appearance parameters are robust and allow for incredible customization. The following images provide examples of appropriate clinical appearance, inappropriate clinical appearance, and the sort of avatar appearance that students could create without provided institutional guidance and boundary setting for student appearance in virtual worlds.

Over time, norms associated with appearance for clinical appearance have changed. Many reading this text remember the days of nursing caps and capes. Today's expectations are perhaps more liberal, but the point is that modeled behavior in virtual environments should be consistent with real-world educational and clinical environments. This is important from several perspectives related to acculturation. Students learn from the professional affinity groups they hope to join. Identifying with one's future affinity group is an important tenet of learning (Bauman, 2010; Bauman & Games, 2011; Games & Bauman, 2011; Gee, 2003).

Navigating institutional expectations as well as social and professional mores in virtual worlds can be confusing, particularly when the original purpose of existing commercial platforms like *Second Life* or *World of Warcraft* are designed for social networking and entertainment, rather than clinical and professional education. Teachers and administrators should consider how they would react to inappropriate in-world behavior and appearance. Consider the following unfolding narrative

> . . . if a student's avatar is dressed in a manner inconsistent with institution policy, consequences should be accurately and concurrently situated within the context of both the virtual and real worlds. Put simply, if professional attire is required when seeing patients in clinic, then the virtual clinic should adhere to the same rules. One can imagine how lessons in professional conduct related to character appearance and behavior could be further situated in a number of contexts. For example, should players in the virtual world fail to adhere to expected personal protective precautions, they may have a significant exposure, leading to illness. In this way, a violation of policy becomes another facet of learning rather than a punitive consequence related to the inexperience of a novice learner.
>
> —*Bauman, p. 202*

When policies related to *in-world* behavior and appearance are well thought out and clearly communicated, they move beyond supporting lesson plans and objectives and become an integral part of the learning.

The malleability of players' avatars and NPCs (Non-Player Characters) also provides an important opportunity for instructors to address cultural diversity that does not exist in real-world, homogeneous learning populations. The topic of cultural diversity is more fully discussed in Chapter 7, but is worth introducing here in the context of acculturation and the preparation of nursing students for clinical practice. Many students complete nursing school among populations that largely mirror the student body. For instance, in many nursing schools the students and faculty are predominantly white and female. Yet these students in many cases are going to transition into practice environments with diverse patient and professional populations.

When designed using frameworks like the ecology of culturally competent design, virtual world encounters can be designed to provide authentic cultural experiences. These sorts of in-world experiences provide first contact opportunities in controlled environments where experiences can be adequately debriefed. The importance of debriefing must be emphasized when designing and facilitating experiences focusing on culture and diversity, because the topic is often new to some students and can lead to important discursive, sometimes emotionally charged discussions that will shape future practice (Bauman, 2010; Bauman & Games, 2011; Games & Bauman, 2011).

Consistency

Game-based and virtual worlds provide a level of consistency not available with other types of clinical environments. Cases or scenarios presented in a fixed mannikin-based simulation laboratory have the advantage of allowing students to work through the same case numerous times or to take a "do-over" to remediate performance after receiving feedback from peers and facilitators during debriefings. This is of course also possible in a digital environment. However, the same cases or scenarios presented in the fixed mannikin-based simulation laboratories often unfold differently based on who is facilitating the session, even when scenario guidelines and objectives are provided to facilitators and supervising faculty. This variable is not always negative—but can be confusing to students with less or no clinical experience and limited experience in the laboratory setting.

The digital setting can be designed so that it is completely automated. A video game can provide a narrative and environment that provides consistent feedback and responses for all students over time. Further, game-based experiences can allow students to "level-up" to encounter more challenging in-game experiences based on objective-driven accomplishments. This is not to say that instructors cannot enter the environment to introduce additional variables to scenarios but instructors should be aware that unmapped and untested variables can significantly alter narratives existing in virtual worlds, just as they do in real-world clinical settings.

For example, having a parent or spouse enter a patient's room during a history and physical can significantly change the outcome of the patient–clinician encounter. Similarly, the presence, particularly the unexpected appearance, of another player character in an environment will change the outcome of the unfolding narrative taking place in the game-based digital environment, especially if that player character is known to be an instructor.

Just as facilitators and instructors are advised to avoid breaking the fidelity of mannikin-based simulation scenarios, they also should avoid breaking the fidelity of digital environments. Let narratives play out; provide environmental cues or just-in-time information to redirect and move narratives forward. Learning ceases to be experimental, even when leveraging simulation and game-based technology, when teachers handhold and micro-manage learning taking place in created environments. Breaks in fidelity should be limited to learner safety and those circumstances where students lose their way to the extent that it is difficult for them to regroup and move toward lesson objectives.

All of this said, it is important to recognize that the created environment, mannikin or digitally based, by its very nature allows and encourages students to contribute to their own learning. Instructors will find that with experience they will be able to predict how and when students will interact with their environment and others present in the environment. This will add richness to learning. It will allow teachers to understand how students can get to very dangerous places for very good reasons. The perils that we sometimes find students in are sometimes directly related to the inconsistency we inject into otherwise clear learning scenarios.

Best Practices

Nursing is a discipline known for following best practices, particularly as it relates to facilitating patient care (Closs & Cheater, 1999). Explaining best practices or having students read about them provides them with didactic information. Maintaining a robust reading practice within a clinical field is essential for safe, up-to-date clinical practice. This said, it can be difficult for clinical instructors to model best practices in actual clinical environments for various reasons.

While best practices are often reported in the scholarly literature, until students develop familiarity with basic practice standards it is difficult for them to understand best practices to the extent that they can adequately apply them to any given clinical site or encounter. Further, best practices are by their very nature a moving target. For example, hyperventilation was thought to be not only a lifesaving practice during cardiac resuscitation, it was considered best practice. We now understand that hyperventilation during cardiac arrest actually decreases survival and can increase postresuscitation complications. Current best practice limits the rate and volume of ventilations during resuscitation efforts (Kellum, Kennedy, & Ewy, 2006). What was once considered best practice is now in direct contradiction to current best practice.

Because best practices are driven by science, and technology has accelerated the process of scientific discovery, curriculums and the textbooks used to support best practices find it difficult to remain current. Further, students may not have the opportunity to engage current best practices while such practices are still current. In this sense the lag time in the traditional way curricula are designed and supported have the potential to prepare students for types of practices that no longer exist in the workplace they are soon to enter.

Digital environments are malleable by nature and with proper support are more agile than didactic tools used to support clinical education. We can introduce emerging and best practices to pre-licensure students as they occur. Further, licensed professionals can engage and explore emerging and defined best practices in digital and fixed-simulation environments at a much more rapid pace. In addition, we can compare older practices to emerging practices using sophisticated computer modeling to test hypotheses to define and reinforce best practices.

Maintenance

Maintenance of any digital tool, whether it is a stand-alone tool or a continuous environment like an MMOG, is essential to the ability to use such tools effectively and consistently. Those familiar with mannikin-based simulation will attest to the time and effort required to develop or adapt industry-supplied scenarios to meet specific curriculum objectives that attend to the variations of institutional practice standards. We must dedicate further resources to the IT and physical maintenance of these tools for them to remain in viable working order. Also, the more we use any tool (a sign of its capabilities) the more time we must dedicate to maintaining the tool.

This paradigm exists and is perhaps exacerbated in virtual environments because virtual environments often evolve and update quickly. As technology standards improve and change, updates for MMOG digital environments are just as important if not more important than the game-based learning existing among stand-alone platforms. For example, if there is a screen-based simulation tool on a discrete computer and this tool is meeting objectives, little if any maintenance is required to sustain this tool as is. However, cloud- or web-based applications and software updates needed to meet new IT specifications will have significant impact on learner access and experience if not maintained regularly. Consider the number of updates now released for smartphone and mobile device applications. Many of these updates for mobile technology and web-based MMOGs are driven by user feedback. The success of digital tools is dependent on their use and the willingness of commercial developers and, in the case of educational venues, and educational designers, to accept feedback from end users in order to foster a sense of continuous quality improvement.

In order to use simulation and game-based technology to prepare students for actual clinical environments, it is important to consider who the end user actually is. The easy answer is that the end user is the student. The complex and comprehensive answer also considers other stakeholders. To a large extent the end user question should first consider the instructors and faculty that are going to facilitate the educational process. Educators will not adopt technology if it is too complicated or time consuming for faculty to use. We discuss this point in more detail in Chapter 6, but it is important and worth emphasizing here. Future employers should also be considered as an end user. We want to take advantage of simulation and game-based learning to prepare students for future work environments. Thus we must select products and create environments that authentically map to these environments and take care to update and maintain these environments so they remain current and authentic. Finally, we must consider the patient as an end user. If we are committed to instilling best practices driven by evidence-based practices (Closs & Cheater, 1999; Grol & Grimshaw, 2003), then what we are really hoping for is to use these environments so that they are translational and transformative. In this context the integration of digital tools into curricula must support educational practices that in turn prepare students for best practices based on evidence that we hope will improve patient outcome.

ROLES FOR GAME-BASED LEARNING: PRIMARY OR PRE-LICENSURE EDUCATION, CONTINUING EDUCATION, AND CLINICAL THREAT ASSESSMENT

Learning is a continuous process. Licensing and accrediting bodies require and recommend topics and length of training for various institutions' clinician practice credentials and certifications. Yet clinical proficiency requires continuing if not continuous education. Few if any clinicians would argue this point. We can use and leverage simulation and game-based learning in various capacities to support areas of learning and discovery, including pre-licensure education, continuing nursing, and other types of clinical education and institutional or context-specific threat assessment.

Primary or Pre-Licensure Education

Pre-licensure education refers to engaging in primary nursing education or other discipline-specific training that occurs before a nurse is admitted to the profession or level of a profession. From this perspective this category includes students entirely new to the profession who are enrolled in baccalaureate and associate degree programs in nursing. It also encompasses graduate-level training preparing existing nurses for new advanced practice roles.

Continuing Education

For the purpose of this discussion, continuing education encompasses training that occurs after license to practice has been granted or training that learners engage in to maintain or attain specific practice status and credentials. Continuing education is often required by licensing boards and can also be employer specific. It is also required to maintain professional credentials such as maintaining status as a Certified Emergence Nurse (CEN) via the Certified Emergency Nurses Association or Critical Care Registered Nurse (CCRN) through the American Association of Critical Care Nurses.

Clinical Threat Assessment and Patient Safety

Disaster exercises using various types of simulation are widely believed to be beneficial in preparing organizations and instuitions for actual disasters (Bartley, Stella, & Walsh, 2006). More recently, simulation is being used to evaluate team interactions and institutional policy that threatens patient safety or negatively impacts patient outcome. From this perspective, simulation, often mannikin-based simulation but also augmented reality and sophisticated modeling, is being used to evaluate operational processes within organizations that represent situational threats that impact patient outcome or increase institutional liability. Information gleaned from threat assessment simulation should be used to drive institutional policy (Hamman, 2004).

Simulation and digital modeling within virtual environments can also provide valuable information about anticipated events. For example, in situ simulation or modeled simulation in virtual or created spaces can provide valuable information about how real people will process and execute actual clinical encounters during day-to-day operations and crisis situations. For example, before a new emergency room opens for actual patient care, in situ simulation designed to evaluate low-incidence, high-risk encounters can be designed as an educational threat assessment. This is the institutional equivalent of a dry run or scrimmage. This sort of exercise is formative and may serve to reinforce or change policy and practice guidelines.

The educational facet of the experience will serve to orient staff to a new environment and perhaps new equipment. The threat assessment facet of this exercise evaluates how the team of clinicians interacts in the environment to manage patient care. This type of assessment need not be relegated to crisis management or low-incidence, high-risk event preparation, but can also be used to evaluate, establish, and refine policies and protocols that shape the day-to-day interactions of staff working within a given environment. From a broader perspective, the use of simulation (regardless of type) as an assessment tool transcends and moves beyond discrete task and behavioral training for individual learners and even teams of clinicians found in clinical care settings and becomes a translational opportunity to inform institutional and public policy (Gaba, 2004).

DESIGN CASE STUDY: MICRO SCENARIO BASED LEARNING (SBL) FOR AN ONLINE RN TO BSN PROGRAM

One of the key challenges of healthcare education for both degree seekers and professionals engaged in continuing education is the need for learners to master both clinical procedural knowledge and situated practices in order to prepare for work in the field. The Micro Scenario Based Learning (Micro-SBL) tool in development at University of Wisconsin–Extension for University of

Wisconsin – Green Bay's online RN to BSN program (BSN-LINC) offers one example of how interactive simulations and games can be used to confront this challenge in healthcare education. This case will offer a perspective on the essential challenges and opportunities presented by the BSN-LINC program, and the design path taken by the team at UW-Extension to meet the instructional needs of the online learners in this program.

Like many online learning initiatives, BSN-LINC is based on a successful face-to-face instructional program. The model of porting traditional instruction to online or blended instruction always carries with it certain challenges. While some of these challenges are tied to marketing or student expectations, others are tied to the unique constraints and affordances of online teaching and learning. This is especially true for programs like those granting nursing degrees that are concerned with preparing learners for a field where interpersonal skills and situated understandings are at least as important as technical skills and domain knowledge (Lockyer, Sargeant, Curran, & Fleet, 2006).

One essential element in a practitioner-oriented distance education program like BSN-LINC that can offset some of the challenges introduced by geographic barriers is the provision of practicum experiences with partner organizations. Practicum courses are an expected and essential element in nursing education programs. However, they include the challenges that are present in any form of inter-institutional collaboration. Different organizations have different institutional norms. The presence of conflicting personality types among participants can increase as more people are added in inter-institutional collaboration. Further, administrative and even legal regulations have the capacity to increase substantially when organizations collaborate.

A distance-based practicum component, especially one like BSN-LINC, which focuses on out of state students, likely involves many of these complicating factors. In particular, increased difficulty coordinating with partner institutions, and more variability and difficulty facilitating practicum experiences have been notable challenges for the BSN-LINC program (Vandenhouten & Block, 2005). Challenges like these increase the need and desire of the teaching institutions to offer learners additional immersive resources to supplement what can be the least consistent aspects of the program.

The micro-SBL system is designed to have utility for more than just BSN-LINC courses, yet it offers a clear example of how a simulation or game-based tool can create a greater level of consistency of instructional experiences among geographically dispersed nursing students. In the case of the micro-SBL tool, the focus is specifically on taking case-based learning materials that are used in face-to-face instruction and effectively transforming them into meaningful experiences for students to use independently in an e-Learning environment. The expectation that instructors will debrief these learning experiences with online students exists. Any micro-SBL should stand on its own as a substantive learning opportunity that captures the complexity of the case on which it is based. The aim of the instructional design team creating this tool was more than simply the creation of individual micro-SBLs for the BSN-LINC program, but the creation of a system that makes it easier for both subject matter experts (SMEs) and developers to generate micro-SBLs based on existing materials for a wide range of programs. Achieving these objectives required close collaboration between SMEs from UW–Green Bay and designers and developers at UW–Extension.

The process began with a faculty member from UW–Green Bay providing a sample clinical case that has previously been used in face-to-face and online courses in the nursing program. Thoughts about how such a case might be implemented online were also provided. Designers and developers at UW-Extension analyzed the case with a focus on how the unique capacities of SBL could improve the learning experience. This meant determining what the generic elements of the case were that would need to be represented in an SBL experience, and focusing on ways in which the experience represented in the case materials could be modified to fit a digitally facilitated instructional experience where no live instructor would be present to respond to learner decisions as they happened.

One of the earliest choices made by the design team was to focus on a tool for micro scenarios that could be played from start to finish in five to ten minutes. This was in response to the initial case provided by the SME and consideration of other cases used in the context of professional education. This contrasts with traditional case scenarios that might take an hour or even a day to complete. Several factors drove this decision:

1. First, as with many cases assembled for professional learning, the contents of the sample case had already been broken down into several distinct segments. This existing division of content seemed to lend itself to smaller SBL experiences.
2. Second, as noted previously, the developers' primary aim wasn't to simply make a single media rich interactive scenario. Rather, the developers hoped to develop a system for creating scenarios that would guide faculty and other SMEs toward collaboration with instructional designers and developers in the future. Based on their extensive experiences working with faculty across the University of Wisconsin system, the UW-Extension team recognized that breaking the intended learning experience into smaller more manageable chunks of content would significantly ease the process of providing content and feedback for their busy faculty counterparts.
3. Finally, and perhaps most importantly, the developers wanted decisions that learners made in a scenario to be meaningful, but also wanted to ensure that the decisions didn't result in unreasonable development requirements for individual scenarios.

The developers' aim to keep scenario development contained is worth considering in greater depth. The most traditional method for creating interactive narrative content for both educational and entertainment purposes involves the use of branching narrative structures. With a branching narrative, the player is offered a choice in response to a prompt and depending on the selection the player makes, they are directed to a specific scene where the consequences of their decision play out. This structure is familiar to anyone who has ever read a *Choose Your Own Adventure*® or other "game book." If you've experienced this form of content, you are likely aware of the fundamental issues that exist in the creation and use of branching narratives.

The largest problem with the branching narrative approach is the tendency for outcomes to multiply exponentially. The common work-around for this problem is to create nodes that funnel back various choices. This diminishes the amount of complexity that emerges with successive choices. However, it creates a second issue: ensuring that user choices are authentic and lead to unique and meaningful outcomes (Gordon, 2004). While the initial case provided for the UW–Extension team didn't require any branching as presented by the SME, the developers were keenly aware of the potential requirement to create alternate outcomes, as this is one of the key features that scenario-based learning experiences can provide. By focusing on a tool for creating micro scenarios, the developers saw a way to limit the amount of branching that could potentially take place in a scenario without directing users back to common nodes that undermine the significance of their decisions. This decision had the helpful additional outcome of limiting the range of content that SMEs would have to generate when transforming a traditional case into a series of micro-SBLs.

The second major design decision the UW–Extension developers made involved cataloging the types of interactions learners would need to make at decision points within a scenario. Based on the materials provided by their faculty counterpart, the developers cataloged the following input types that were required for the first case: multiple-choice, multiple select, and short answer. Short answer decisions might be independent in a case, or they might be tied to a multiple-choice or multiple select question. For instance, the learner might be asked to diagnose a patient's condition based on the symptoms they selected through one of the other answer methods presented earlier in the scenario.

You might note that this list of student decision input methods provided by the SME looks suspiciously like the item types used for a test or other type of assessment, like a survey. The developers were consciously aware of the input methods for student decision making and took two measures to enhance the narrative style of the SBL experience. First, they established a content convention whereby the framing material for these various types of interaction would be written in a narrative format to enhance immersion. Second, rather than providing immediate corrective feedback based on learner decisions in a scenario, they offloaded feedback from the interactions to the end of the scenario so that learners could continue with the scenario despite having made a clinical error.

Students later receive detailed feedback on each step at the conclusion of the scenario. This style of feedback is more closely aligned with experiential learning methodology and debriefing activities used in case-based learning.

Since the initial case did not include branching narratives, the developers provided indirect feedback via interaction with a fictional head nurse who could offer corrective cues to keep the scenario from branching while still allowing the learner to make choices throughout the scenario. Although this may diminish the perception of meaningful choices for learners in the scenario, it offered a way to use the first case as a starting point for developing a micro-SBL scenario authoring system without extending and complicating the development process by focusing too myopically on the conditions of any particular case.

In order to meet other types of conditions for future scenario design not included in the initial case, the developers also created an inventory system for the micro-SBL tool. Drawing inspiration from video game design, as learners proceed through a scenario they can gather various resources and add them to their virtual inventory. Some items in the player's inventory are general resources that can be referenced at any time rather than only during a relevant decision point. This reinforces the importance of cognitive aides during real practice and the ability to access information in real time to support decision making. Other items are tied to a specific scenario and can only be used when the player has access to them in that scenario. While the first prototype features relatively static versions of these items (for example, CT scan image and static patient chart), the tool has been built so that future scenarios will allow SMEs and designers to provide the learner with choices based not only on their grasp of didactic content, but also their capacity to work more dynamically with virtual representations of real-world resources like charts and laboratory findings.

The collaborating faculty member for this project also included references for outside resources, including a medical reference website in the original materials for the case. This prompted the developers to account for two types of inventory items: scenario items like patient charts and other elements that are tied to the specific scenario and information resources that are either real-world resources healthcare professionals use in actual clinical practice or modified versions of such resources that represent real tools that clinicians have access to. Inclusion of informational resources allows developers and SMEs to help learners familiarize themselves with digital tools that contemporary healthcare professionals rely on in real practice, while creating a data architecture that includes scenario resources that lay the groundwork for the development of more deeply interactive micro-SBLs in the future.

Next steps in the implementation of the micro-SBL system by the UW-Extension division of Continuing Education Outreach and e-Learning (CEOEL) include user testing and analysis. Developers will modify the micro-SBL system based on user feedback gleaned from user testing and integrate it into the BSN-LINC curriculum. While the micro-SBL system does not offer the same depth of experience provided by some types of immersive simulation environments, its designers created a system that provides a simple process to make meaningful simulation-based experiences that support practicum elements and more costly and complex immersive simulations.

SUMMARY

This chapter has discussed how we can use virtual reality and game-based learning environments to prepare learners for actual practice settings. The chapter began with a discussion of different types of created spaces included mannikin-based simulation laboratories, virtual and game-based environments, and augmented reality.

The chapter then argued that educators should consider simulation as clinical education and provided a discussion of how and why this argument has merit. Several examples of how simulation supporting and supplementing actual real-world or traditional clinical hours recommendations and requirements both nationally and internationally were discussed.

We also encouraged readers to rethink the relevance and context of learning spaces. We discussed the relevance of fidelity, suspension of disbelief, and theatrics when using modern multimedia teaching spaces. Both environmental and psychological fidelity were defined and the role that they both play on the suspension of disbelief was discussed. We also discussed the importance and role that theatrics should play during simulations taking place in physical and virtual spaces.

Access to virtual environments was addressed from the perspective of safety, acculturation, consistency, best practices, and maintenance. The chapter addressed the importance of the psychological or emotional safety of students who are immersed in simulations and game-based activities. Using digital spaces for acculturation learning activities was also discussed from the perspectives of professional development and the introduction of cultural learning opportunities. We also discussed how simulation and game-based learning can be used to define, explore, and support best practices. The importance of continuous quality improvement and environmental maintenance also was emphasized, stressing that poorly maintained technology is often unused and of little value to any curriculum.

Finally, we documented an in-depth case study focusing on the Micro Scenario Based Learning (SBL) tool developed and implemented in an online RN to BSN program. This tool aims to provide interactive simulations and games that can be used to confront this challenge in healthcare education, specifically nursing healthcare education occurring at a distance through e-Learning platforms.

REFERENCES

Armstrong, M. L., Gessner, B. A., & Skott Cooper, S. (2000). Pots, Pans, Pearls: The nursing professions rich history with distance education for a new century of nursing. *The Journal of Continuing Education in Nursing, 31*(2), 63–70.

Azuma, R. T. (1997). A survey of augmented reality. *Presence: Teleoperators & Virtual Environments, 6*(4), 355.

Azuma, R. T., Baillot, Y, Behringer, R., Feiner, S., Julier, S., & MacIntrye, B. (2001). Recent advances in augmented reality. *IEEE Computer Graphics and Applications, 21*(6), 34–37.

Bartley, B. H., Stella, J. B., & Walsh, L. D. (2006). What a disaster?! Assessing utility of simulated disaster exercise and educational process for improving hospital preparedness. *Prehospital and Disaster Medicine, 21*(4), 249–255.

Bauman, E. (2007). *High fidelity simulation in healthcare*. PhD dissertation, The University of Wisconsin – Madison, United States. Dissertations & Theses @ CIC Institutions database. (Publication no. AAT 3294196 ISBN: 9780549383109 ProQuest document ID: 1453230861)

Bauman, E. (2010). Virtual reality and game-based clinical education. In K. B. Gaberson, & M. H. Oermann (Eds.), *Clinical teaching strategies in nursing education* (3rd ed.). New York, Springer Publishing Company.

Bauman, E. B., & Games, I. A. (2011). Contemporary theory for immersive worlds: Addressing engagement, culture, and diversity. In A. Cheney, & R. Sanders (Eds.), *Teaching and Learning in 3D Immersive Worlds: Pedagogical models and constructivist approaches*. IGI Global.

Boulet, J. R., & Murray, D. R. (2010). Requirements for practical implementation. *Anesthesiology, 112*(4), 1041–1051.

Closs, S. J., & Cheater, F. M. (1999). Evidence for nursing practice: A clarification of the issues. *Journal of Advanced Nursing, 30*(1), 10–17.

Dieckmann, P., Gaba, D., & Rall, M. (2007). Deepening the theoretical foundations of patient simulation as social practice. *Simulation in Healthcare, 2*(3), 183–193.

Erickson, P. M., Fox, W. S., & Stewart, D. (Eds.). (2010). National standards for teachers of family and consumer sciences: Research, implementation, and resources. Published electronically by National Association of Teacher Educators for Family and Consumer Sciences. Available at http://natefacs.org/JFCSE/Standards_eBook/Standards_eBook.pdf

Faragher, J. F., Boese, T., Decker, S., & Sando, C. (2011). Standards of best practice: Simulation. *Simulation in Nursing, 7*(4), S1–S20.

Flanagan, B., Nestel, D., & Joseph, M. (2004). Making patient safety the focus: Crisis resource management in the undergraduate curriculum. *Medical Education, 38*(1), 56–66.

Friedrich, M. J. (2002). Practice makes perfect: Risk-free medical training with patient simulators. *Jama, 288*(22), 2808, 2811–2812.

Gallagher, C. J., & Tan, J. M. (2010). The current status of simulation in the maintenance of certification in anesthesia. *International Anesthesiology Clinics, 48*(3), 83–99.

Gaba, D. M. (2004). The future vision of simulation in health care. *Quality and Safety in Health Care, 13*(Suppl. 1), i2–i10.

Gamage, J., Tretiakov, A., & Crump, B (2011). Teacher perceptions of learning affordances of multi-user virtual environments. *Computers & Education, 57*(4), 2406–2413.

Games, I., & Bauman, E. (2011) Virtual worlds: An environment for cultural sensitivity education in the health sciences. *International Journal of Web Based Communities 7*(2), 189–205, doi: 10.1504/IJWBC.2011.039510.

Gee, J. P. (2003). *What videogames have to teach us about learning and literacy.* New York, NY: Palgrave-McMillan.

Glavin, R. J., & Maran, N. J. (2003). Integrating human factors into the medical curriculum. *Medical Education, 37*(Suppl. 1), 59–64.

Gordon, A. (2004) Authoring Branching Storylines for Training Applications. Proceedings of the Sixth International Conference of the Learning Sciences (ICLS-04). Santa Monica, CA, June 22–26.

Gordon, J. A., Oriol, N. E., & Cooper, J. B. (2004). Bringing good teaching cases "to life": A simulator-based medical education service. *Academic Medicine, 79*(1), 23–27.

Gore, T., Van Gele, P., Ravert, P., & Mabire, C. (2012). A 2010 Survey of the INACSL Membership about Simulation Use. *Clinical Simulation in Nursing, 8*(4), E125–E133.

Grol, R., & Grimshaw, J. (2003). From best evidence to best practice: effective implementation of change in patients' care. *The Lancet, 336,* 1225–1230.

Halamek, L. P., Kaegi, D. M., Gaba, D. M., Sowb, Y. A., Smith, B. C., Smith, B. E. et al. (2000). Time for a new paradigm in pediatric medical education: Teaching neonatal resuscitation in a simulated delivery room environment. *Pediatrics, 106*(4), E45.

Hamman, W. R. (2004). The complexity of team training: what we have learned from aviation and its applications to medicine. *Quality Safety Health Care, 13*(Supplemental 1), i72–i179.

Hayden, J. (2010). Use of simulation in nursing education: National survey results. *Journal of nursing regulation, 1*(3), 53–57.

Issenberg, S. B., & Scalese, R. J. (2008). Simulation in health care education. *Perspectives in Biology and Medicine, 51*(1), 31–46.

Kellum, M. J., Kennedy, K. W., & Ewy, G. A. (2006). Cardiocerebral resuscitation improves survival of patients in out-of-hospital cardiac arrest. *The Journal American Journal of Medicine, 119*(4), 335–340.

Kneebone, R. L., Scott, W., Darzi, A., & Horrocks, (2004). Simulation and clinical practice: strengthening the relationship, *Medical Education, 38*(10), 1095–1102.

Lane, J. L., Slavin, S., & Ziv, A. (2001). Simulation in medical education: A review. *Simulation & Gaming, 32*(3), 297–314.

Leighton, K., & Dubas, J. (2009). Simulated death: An innovative approach to teaching ennd-of-life care. *Clinical Simulation in Nursing, 5*(6), e223–e230.

Lockyer, J., Sargeant, J., Curran, P., & Fleet, L. (2006). The transition from face-to-face to online CME facilitation. *Medical Teacher, 28*(7), 625–630.

Nursing Midwifery Council. (2007). Nursing and Midwifery Council Circular, *36*(2007), United Kingdom.

Seropian, M. A. (2003). General concepts in full scale simulation: Getting started. *Anesthesia and Analgesia, 97*(6), 1695–1705.

Shapiro, M. J., & Simmons, W. (2002). High fidelity medical simulation: a new paradigm in medical education. *Med Health RI*, *85*(10), 316–317.

Society for Simulation in Healthcare. (2012). SSH Accreditation Process. Informational Guide for the Accreditation Process from the SSH Council for Accreditation of Healthcare Simulation Programs.

Sperlazza, E., & Cangelosi, P. R. (2009). The power of pretend: Using simulation to teach end of life care. *Nurse Educator*, *34*(6), 276–280.

Stewart, L. (1992). Ethical issues in postexperimental and postexperiential debriefing. *Simulation and Gaming*, *23*(2), 196–211.

Thiagarajan, S. (1992). Using games for debriefing. *Simulation and Gaming*, *23*(2), 161–173.

Utah Administrative Code, Nurse Practice Act, Rule R156-31b, Section E, Sub ii. Accessed electronically 01/15/2012.

Vandenhouten, C., & Block, D. (2005). A case study of a distance-based public health nursing/community health nursing practicum. *Public Health Nursing*, *22*(2), 166–171.

Wisconsin Department of Health Services, WMS Section (2011). Wisconsin Standardized Paramedic Curriculum.

Ziv, A., Wolpe, P. R., Small, S. D., & Glick, S. (2003). Simulation-based medical education: An ethical imperative. *Academic Medicine*, *78*(8), 783–788.

6

Fitting Virtual Reality and Game-Based Learning Into an Existing Curriculum

PENNY RALSTON-BERG AND MIGUEL LARA

INTRODUCTION

*T*echnology is an ongoing critical external contextual factor that influences the content, teaching-learning strategies, and course management of nursing curricula (Iwasiw, Goldenberg, & Andrusyszyn, 2005). Different technologies offer certain capabilities that make it more appropriate for certain learning experiences than others (Kozma, 1994). When educators consider the addition of virtual reality and game-based learning to an existing curriculum, they must assess both to determine if and how they will have the most positive impact on learning. Without prior analysis and thoughtful, appropriate, purposeful implementation aligned with learning objectives, virtual reality and game-based learning can become a distraction or worse yet a barrier to learning. For instance, it would be very difficult for nurses to learn to perform various procedural aspects of nursing like IV therapy or wound care just by listening to lectures via podcast or broadcast through radio. On the other hand, normal-size 3-D anatomy models might provide a better spatial reference than a black and white drawing.

MAXIMIZING IMPACT

The proper fit of any technology, including digital games and virtual environments, within a curriculum is in direct relation to the extent in which the integration of the technology makes a teaching-learning strategy more *effective*, *efficient*, and *appealing*. In other words, what impact does the game or virtual environment have on learning? Is the technology reasonably efficient based on the teaching situation, and is it appealing enough to students to maintain engagement and motivation through the learning process?

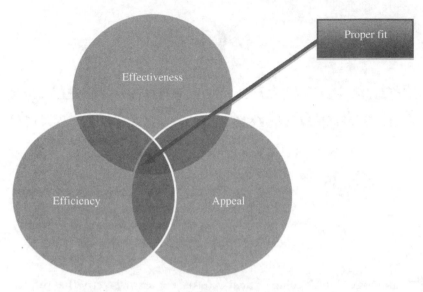

FIGURE 6.1
Model for determining curricular fit

To have a truly good fit, all three indicators should be equally balanced. In other words, even though a digital game can be highly alluring and engaging it will not be a good curricular fit if students are not learning the intended concepts or skills. Likewise a virtual environment based strictly on content delivery without sufficient activities to engage and challenge the learner does not have a high enough impact on learning to justify the added time and costs associated with setting up such an environment (Figure 6.1).

As shown in Figure 6.1, the three quality indicators (effectiveness, efficiency, and appeal) can guide us in the selection of a game-based or virtual environment learning interventions with a proper curricular fit.

Effectiveness

We measure the effectiveness of an instructional strategy in relation to the goals and objectives of the instruction (Reigeluth & Merrill, 1979), and the accuracy, comprehensiveness, and freshness of the content (Weston, McAlpine, & Bordonaro, 1995). When determining effectiveness to maximize impact, ask the following questions regarding the effectiveness of using games and virtual spaces for learning:

• Is the use of the game or virtual space aligned with the learning objectives of the specific instructional section?

- Are the general characteristics of the target students known?
- Do the target students have the practice time, skills, and prior knowledge to enable them to interact with the game or virtual space?
- Will the students' interaction with the game or virtual space facilitate acquiring the intended knowledge or mastery of the intended skills?
- Will the knowledge acquired in the game or virtual space transfer properly to real situations?

When considering good curricular fit, virtual reality and game-based learning must be aligned to learning objectives and desired outcomes. We must clearly define objectives and outcomes early in the process in order to select the most appropriate game or virtual reality experience. In some cases, after clarifying objectives and outcomes, it may become evident that games or virtual environments are not the best solution for the situation at hand. Other more traditional methods may make a more positive impact on learning without the use of virtual reality or game-based learning.

One approach to determine a good curricular fit is to translate the learning objectives or desired outcomes into key functions. In terms of distance learning, Aldrich (2009a) suggests that virtual worlds are most appropriate for social, diversity, or community-related activities. For example, virtual worlds can add feelings of proximity, emotional connection, and social presence to a group of distance students working together to complete a team-based activity. Virtual communities where members share a common interest can increase the sense or feeling of community among students and allow them to practice skills with others.

Aldrich (2009a) also suggests that games and simulations can be strategically added to a course to increase student engagement. Aldrich argues that games must be matched to the specific needs and the flow of the course in order to be used effectively. For example, in the context of nursing, a quick fun game could be added to help bring lightness to a dense lecture. Or material difficult to comprehend in a text-based format could be transformed to a challenging simulation. Both examples use games to overcome different types of challenges to student learning.

Virtual worlds or digital environments as stand-alone learning environments are only effective when they offer some form of engagement that maps back to curriculum objectives. For lessons targeting objectives that normally occur in face-to-face labs, Aldrich recommends adding stand-alone digital simulation or using other game or simulation-based experiences to supplement a virtual world (2009a). In other words, game-based activities should exist within virtual spaces that support lesson objectives.

Virtual worlds on their own can be empty and without inherent instructional purpose unless specific social events, environments, or simulations are added to them. Simulations allow learners to use virtual models, tools, instruments, equipment, and processes in a reality-based environment.

Some environments also allow students to be creators of their own content and simulations. Aldrich (2009a) describes simulations as being most appropriate for nonlinear, dynamic content where learners are asked to quickly analyze and make decisions based on ever-changing environmental situations. In terms of nursing education, this applies to practices that require critical decision making and implementation of effective practice—skills that learners will use in real-world clinical environments after a class is completed.

Virtual Worlds and Communication

Multi-user virtual environments (MUVE), or virtual worlds, allow users to meet and interact in-world through their avatars. An avatar is a customized digital graphic representation of oneself. In most virtual worlds, avatars can communicate with each other through text-based chat and predefined nonverbal gestures. There are a few virtual worlds, like *Second Life*, that have introduced voice features to allow verbal communication.

According to the media richness theory (Daft and Lengel, 1986), the richer the media, that is the more communication channels and cues are used, the more effective the communication. In virtual worlds, media richness influences the level of "co-presence," or the extent to which users feel they are together in the same place (Wadley, Gibbs, & Ducheneaut, 2009).

Visual cues such as avatar gaze and body gestures promote the sense of social presence. For instance, avatar gaze can indicate the direction in which a user is looking and direct attention to other users toward an object of interest (Montoya, Massey, & Lockwood, 2011) while body gestures can express the feelings or emotions of users.

Johnson, Vorderstrasse, and Shaw (2009) discuss an example of a nursing program that uses a virtual world as a communication space. Duke University School of Nursing students use *Second Life* to attend lectures in a building that resembles an actual existing real-world teaching space. The virtual classrooms include a podium from which the instructor lectures while the students' avatars sit in virtual chairs. PowerPoint presentations are displayed on a whiteboard and a blackboard is used for students to post questions. Several nursing informatics students were surveyed about their perceptions of learning, and their self-rated gains in content within three different environments: a learning management system, webinars, and the *Second Life* virtual world. The results showed that "Second Life was significantly higher than that of a learning management system for overall assessment of the learning environment and perceived quality of instruction. Students reported that having class in Second Life helped to clarify class content and found the class discussions more spontaneous" (Johnson et al. 2009, p. 5).

Johnson et al. (2009) recognize that teaching in the virtual world presents some challenges that can be mitigated by providing a proper introduction and orientation to virtual worlds being used as teaching spaces. Students should be encouraged and allowed to become familiar with virtual environments. Students need to understand the basics of in-world navigation, interaction, and communication before they are tasked with more complex lessons supporting curriculum objectives. Furthermore, Johnson et al. (2009) argue that sessions held in the virtual world complement the combination of more common and traditional instructional modalities. Technology like virtual environments should support and enhance instructional approaches like Web 2.0 technologies (blogs, wikis, podcasts) and if possible by holding regular face-to-face meetings. As previously discussed and emphasized throughout this text we must adequately prepare students to use and interact within virtual spaces and have appropriate debriefing activities to promote reflection and discussion of the virtual experience.

Games and Simulations

The games and virtual spaces literature continues to exemplify successful instances of game and virtual reality integration into nursing curricula. Indeed, the use of games has been explored in nursing education even prior to the digital era. Wolf and Duffy (1979) provide several examples of non-digital games appropriate for psychiatric nursing including the *Assignment Game*, developed by John Wiley and Sons, which encourages decision making by simulating actual patient situations and assignments for nursing students; and *HOSPITEX: Hospital Ward Management Exercise* developed by Didactic Systems where players take the role of a head nurse in a hospital and practice making decisions under pressure.

More recently, emerging technologies such as high-resolution 3-D digital animation have promoted the design and development of effective and very appealing games and virtual spaces. For example, Stanford University Medical Media created a 3-D virtual emergency department where students assume the roles of a nurse, X-ray technician, or an emergency room physician in six trauma scenarios. According to the creators of this virtual environment, the 3-D virtual emergency department has the potential to enhance leadership, cooperation, and communication skills that can be transferred from the virtual environment to actual real-world clinical environments (Raths, 2006). The ability to transfer the knowledge acquired in the game or virtual space to a real situation is characteristic of a good curricular fit.

Virtual environments and simulations are conducive as an ideal space for experiential learning to occur. Experiential learning refers to the active process of learning by doing, that is, learning from the experience of actually having done something as opposed to only having passively listened to it or read it. According to Kolb (1975) a concrete experience is the major source of learning; the concrete experience is followed by additional steps to reinforce learning: (1) observing and reflecting upon that experience, (2) forming abstract concepts based upon the reflection, and (3) testing the new concepts.

Experiential learning or learning by doing has been widely used in nursing education. In nursing, learning by doing follows an apprenticeship model in which students learn while working in a hospital or other clinical setting under the supervision of a competent professional mentor. The main limitations of the apprenticeship model include the lack of control over the cases that a nursing student will get exposed to and the minimal feedback often provided to students from their mentors, either for lack of availability or knowledge (Mili, Barr, Harris, & Pittiglio, 2008). Computer simulations can provide a convenient and consistent way for nursing students to engage in deliberate practice in rare or complex cases they are not exposed to during mentored clinical training.

Simulations require strategic thinking and problem solving while moving the learner through increasingly complex and evolving situations (Bonk & Zhang, 2008). Simulations "use rigorously structured scenarios carefully designed to develop specific competencies that can be directly transferred into the real world" (Aldrich, 2009b, p. 1). The use of simulation-based education originated at NASA in the late 1970s in order to achieve safe flight operations by reducing the human errors in airline accidents (Fanning & Gaba, 2009). Today, simulation-based education is part of all areas of the U.S. military (navy, air force, and army) and has started to be implemented in health sciences as well.

In healthcare, the main application of simulations aims to improve the education and training of clinicians by helping them acquire new knowledge and better understand conceptual relations and dynamics (Gaba, 2004). Indeed, simulations have been used in several ways in nursing schools for more than a century. In the late 1800s nursing schools were already using partial and complex task trainers for students to practice psychomotor skills without causing potential discomfort to real patients (Nehring & Lashley, 2010).

Today, computer simulations allow one or a team of students to solve critical incidents occurring among virtual patients. As previously mentioned, virtual worlds can provide an immersive environment to conduct the simulations. An environment is said to be immersive when visitors have the feeling or perception of being part of it. The level of immersion is influenced by the fidelity of the environment as a whole: graphics quality, audio effects, and responses of interaction with objects.

Simulations Within Virtual Worlds

Using the *Second Life* virtual world as a training client, Chodos, Stroulia, and King (2011) created a general digital platform called MeRiTS (Mixed Reality

Training System), which can be used to simulate a variety of healthcare-related scenarios. For instance, in a paramedic training scenario, students have to (a) rescue a male victim from a car accident, (b) transport him to the hospital, and (c) complete a handoff of the patient to the emergency department staff. Each of these three tasks includes several subtasks that as a whole are intended to train students in specific clinical procedures (checking blood pressure, administering medication, and putting the victim on a stretcher) and communication skills (patient handoff and verbal report to emergency department staff).

Chodos et al. (2011) are currently working with students and nursing instructors at the University of Alberta to assess the educational effectiveness of the paramedic training though the use of simulation. Based on their experience in a pilot, they realized the importance of providing students with training in using the *Second Life* interface before participating in the in-world paramedic training scenario. These findings emphasize the importance of basic environment orientation.

Another advantage of using virtual worlds for simulation purposes is that virtual worlds allow the recording of interactions and communication taking place during the learning activity (Garver et al., 2011). In this way, students and instructors can use the recording as part of the debriefing. A debriefing session should always accompany a simulation in order to discuss the events that took place during the simulation, reflect upon the activities conducted, and assimilate new knowledge and skills toward the production of long-lasting learning (Fanning & Gaba, 2007).

Virtual worlds can also be used to provide a visual representation of authentic and fictitious spaces. By using virtual spaces in this way, students do not have to perform specific tasks within the virtual world. Instead they are free to navigate the virtual space while looking at the buildings and objects within them. Spaces found within virtual worlds often include virtual museums, libraries, exhibitions, and galleries. With this method learners can see discrete spaces found in virtual environments as resources and rewards to promote learner engagement and successful learning outcomes. While this sort of free-wheeling exploration can provide interesting exposure and orientation opportunities for participants, the true potential for engagement occurs when these spaces are coupled with activities or in-world games or simulations. Virtual spaces that lack goals or objectives often associated with in-world games and simulations may be aesthetically pleasing but offer limited opportunities for learner engagement and more complex learning.

The Virtual Neurological Education Centre (VNEC) built a virtual space to provide an immersive, interactive experience for learners to become familiar with neurological disabilities and rehabilitation equipment and techniques (Boulos, Hetherington, & Wheeler, 2007). The VNEC environment includes different virtual rooms including a medical and a virtual neurological department. Visitors can navigate this setting and explore and operate virtual replicas

TABLE 6.1
Virtual World Activity Appropriateness Matrix

Type of Activity	Description	Appropriateness
Communication	Virtual office hours, one-to-one communication, or replicated traditional classroom	Less appropriate
	Class discussion or small group communication related to other in-world activities	More appropriate
Presentation	Sharing content through text, visual, audio, or video format	Less appropriate
Observation	Locations or situations not available/accessible in learners' real-world life (e.g., geographic locations, cultures, settings)	More appropriate
Role Play	Activities supporting circumstances outside learners' real-life experience through role play (issues of class, power, ethnicity, gender, mental illness, physical disability, etc.)	More appropriate
Simulation	Simulated planning, analysis, and decision making under pressure of external stressors (healthcare practices, disaster management, dangerous or limited situations)	More appropriate
Immersion	Interaction with content (i.e., walking through human anatomy, experiencing a disaster, virtual testing that guides learners through an anatomical lesson)	More appropriate

of the medical equipment including detailed descriptions and information about their use.

Based on the preceding information and the examples provided, Table 6.1 illustrates different activities in which virtual worlds can be implemented within nursing and other health sciences curricula and their level of appropriateness considering the three quality descriptors of instruction (effectiveness, efficiency, and appeal).

Efficiency

Efficiency, in the context of education, refers to the design, development, and delivery of instruction "in ways that use the least resources for the same or better results" (Januszewski & Molenda, 2008, p. 59). In addition to learning objectives, cost, time, and complexity also influence choice of virtual reality and game-based learning. Figure 6.2 illustrates how learning objectives remain the main consideration in selecting an appropriate technology. Cost represents the financial resources necessary to implement and support a technology. Complexity refers to the fidelity of a technology—be it low fidelity that is relatively easy to implement and use or high fidelity that requires orientation

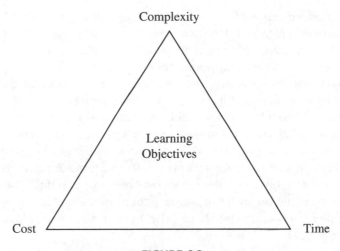

FIGURE 6.2
Considerations for selection of technology

and guidance to use effectively. Time refers to both the time spent in orientation as well as man hours to create, implement, evaluate, and support a technology (Aleckson & Ralston-Berg, 2011).

Several technologies may provide appealing, viable options to effectively meet a set of learning objectives. However, the costs of the technology and time commitment by staff to support it or faculty and students to learn to use it may be beyond the available resources.

As previously discussed, virtual worlds are most appropriate for community-oriented activities or for very focused and specific types of observations and simulations. Using a virtual world for presentation of content to single users or allowing simple interaction in the form of a quizzing tool would not be worth the time, effort, and orientation needed to acquaint learners with the virtual system. Text, audio, video, and simple interactions can be delivered in numerous ways outside the virtual environment.

Observation of dangerous or expensive situations, role-play, simulation and immersion experiences are more appropriate than simple communication or presentation of content for virtual environments. For example, using a virtual world as a platform only for lecturing and displaying presentations might be effective and appealing but there is still the issue of efficiency. The virtual space in *Second Life* (usually called "islands") is not owned by the institution but rented on an annual basis. Moreover, students interacting in environments like *Second Life* need to have computer hardware and broadband Internet access capable enough to run the virtual world application.

In terms of efficiency one must consider whether or not a virtual space is the most appropriate solution for simple communication and lecture. Will the appeal and effectiveness of a novel environment justify the added expense, orientation time, and technical requirements? Viable alternatives might include using conferencing applications, tools available within a course management system, or other institution-supported tools.

Looking specifically at time and cost as they relate to maximizing impact, virtual reality or game-based learning with low instructional impact but high investment of resources is not viable for most situations. As shown in Table 6.2, both low-impact and high-impact learning can occur in low- or no-cost solutions (lower quadrants). A solution does not need to be expensive to have a high impact on learning. However, the more customized, detailed, or complex a solution becomes, the more costs rise (upper right). The quadrant to be avoided is the upper left quadrant where solutions are highly customized, complex, and costly but have little impact on learning (Aleckson & Ralston-Berg, 2011).

Questions to ask regarding the efficiency of using games and virtual environments for learning include:

- How much time and money are needed to design, develop, and use the digital game or virtual space?
- How much additional time will be required to debrief the digital game or virtual space activity?
- How expensive is the type of equipment (hardware and software) that students will need to have in order to access the game or virtual space?
- How many people will need to be concurrently participating when interacting with the digital game or virtual space activity?
- Will the game or virtual space be used in a single course or adapted and repurposed for use in several courses?
- How much time and money will be required to evaluate and revise elements from the game or virtual space?
- Are there any other viable technologies that cost less or require less time and fewer human resources but achieve the same learning objectives?

TABLE 6.2
Time and Cost Related to Instructional Impact

$$$$	High cost, Low impact PowerPoint viewed in virtual world	High cost, High impact High fidelity patient simulator
	Low cost, Low impact Short, interactive quizzes	Low cost, High impact Online decision making simulations
	Low Impact	High Impact

Appeal

Appeal refers to the capacity in which a learning strategy can keep learners' attention and engagement. Well-designed games and virtual spaces have great appeal and are quite motivating. Games are natural tools that can increase learner's intrinsic motivation by providing challenging and engaging activities (Malone & Lepper, 1987).

Appeal is commonly associated with the visual look and feel or cognitive challenge associated with a virtual environment or game-based learning activity. However, it also refers to usability or ease of use of the environment or game. Learners should be able to fully participate in the system without excessive instruction, guidance, or technical support from faculty or staff. When learners find a learning environment difficult to use, they become frustrated and will not actively participate in the instruction. A learning environment that lacks appeal may also be more difficult for faculty to facilitate and manage as part of the learning process.

Questions to ask regarding appeal include:

- Will students find the game or virtual space attractive and interesting?
- Is the game or virtual space motivating?
- Does the game or virtual space present intellectual and motivational challenges?
- Is the interface of the game or virtual space user-friendly and easily navigated?

USE IN COMBINATION WITH OTHER METHODS

When incorporating virtual reality or game-based learning into existing curriculum, it is important to provide a framework or structure for learning activities. As discussed in previous chapters, this structure should include an orientation to the digital or simulation-based environment and practice time and space prior to asking students to actively engage in learning activities. Further, it is important to facilitate a debriefing of activities related to game and simulation orientation. Providing a debriefing of activities that supports orientation to the environment will frame later reflective debriefing processes focused on curriculum objectives (Figure 6.3).

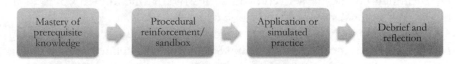

FIGURE 6.3
Framework for integration of virtual reality or game-based learning

Conklin (2007) published examples of *101 Uses of Second Life* in the College Classroom. Most examples show use of virtual environments as a supplement to face-to-face or online education activities. The activities taking place in the virtual environment are focused and related to specific learning objectives. Virtual worlds are rarely the sole delivery method for all aspects of a course. Relative to fit, learning objectives should align throughout the activities in an instructional unit, not just within the virtual reality or game-based learning environment. The designer and instructor of the larger instructional unit should take care to provide transitions and facilitation as students progress through various stages of the larger instructional unit.

For example, in an online course with a unit containing virtual clinical simulation, learners should first be presented with background information and required prerequisite knowledge within the course management system. Students would then receive instructions on how to navigate from the course management system to the simulation as well as expectations and objectives for completing the simulation. At this point it is crucial for students to understand how the simulation fits within the unit. Upon completion of the simulation, students are guided through a debriefing and reflect on their experiences. The debriefing should map back to the objectives for the unit. Sharing objectives and expectations at each step maintains the common thread through all activities within a unit.

CHARACTERISTICS OF E-LEARNING AND VIRTUAL ENVIRONMENTS

Characteristics of e-Learning

Since most multi-user virtual environments (MUVEs) are accessible online they can be suitable for courses that are part of distance education programs. This section describes and differentiates several e-learning terms and provides the defining characteristics of each term. Pitfalls that can occur when using MUVEs in e-learning are also identified.

Generally speaking, e-learning refers to any type of instruction that takes place through the Internet (Pastore, 2002). In other words, it refers to any instruction that occurs via any online application such as video-conferencing tools, web browsers, virtual world applications, and so on. Content designed for e-learning courses is delivered by an instructor (mentor-led courses) or by the instructional system (stand-alone courses).

Web technology is the most common method used to deliver e-learning courses (web-based courses). Allen and Seaman (2011) define online learning as a course where at least 80% of the content is delivered online. These types of courses typically provide no face-to-face meetings and only use technology to connect learners with content and instructors.

In e-learning, "virtual learning environment" is a very broad term used to describe any online information space that has been designed to provide instructional interaction (Dillenbourg, 2000). This interaction can be with a mentor, among other students, or just with the course content itself. There are no constraints for the type of media used. Thus, a set of text-based web pages can be considered a virtual learning environment provided that the information is presented in an organized and meaningful way. Online courses are also considered virtual learning environments.

Most, if not all, online courses taught by academic institutions use applications called "Learning Management Systems" (also known as Content Management Systems) to facilitate the class management and delivery by including and aggregating tools for communication, collaboration, grading, and content access. Examples of Learning Management Systems include products like Desire2Learn, Blackboard, and Moodle.

Characteristics of Virtual Environments

Visual MUVEs or virtual worlds are two- or three-dimensional applications where multiple users can interact in and with the environment. Interaction in contemporary virtual environments often takes place through learners' avatars. Some virtual worlds can be accessed through a web browser. These environments require no additional software. However, some virtual environments like *Second Life* require downloading and installing of proprietary software. It is also important to note that use of virtual environments does not automatically mean interaction or interactivity will take place. Virtual worlds provide only an environment where interaction may take place. Virtual worlds on their own are limited to providing only a means of communication and in some cases the ability to create objects and scenes for use in the world. The most engaging virtual worlds include games, simulations, or other instructional activities added to make them structurally more interactive.

For example, CliniSpace™, a virtual environment produced by Innovation in Learning, Inc. provides custom virtual environments where learners can engage in communication and assessment-based activities. The environment in itself represents authentic clinical spaces, but it is the ability to interact with the environment and the opportunity for learners to process real-time and just-in-time information that drives student engagement and curriculum objectives. The emergency department scenario found in one of CliniSpace™ modules requires learners to access a patient record, examine the NPC patient, order and interpret lab values and diagnostic findings including an abdominal ultrasound.

Aldrich (2009b) describes the similarities and differences among games, simulations, and virtual worlds in terms of environment, goals, structure, and rigor. Both games and simulations occur within some type of virtual world or

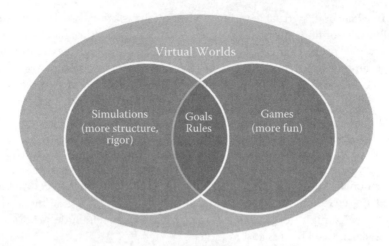

FIGURE 6.4

Similarities and differences of games, simulations, and virtual worlds

environment. While simulations have more defined goals, structure, and rigor to teach specific skills or competencies, games have less stringent goals and constraints. Aldrich also describes games and simulations as needing some sort of community around them to maximize impact. Virtual worlds are described as more social. In other words a stand-alone game or simulation is akin to a stand-alone task trainer. By situating the game or stand-alone simulation (task trainer) within a community or virtual world the skills associated with the task being performed become authentically situated within the professional or clinical context that will occur in actual future practice. For example, many clinical instructors teach IV insertion using an IV arm, a task trainer specifically designed to teach the psychomotor fundamentals of IV insertion. This form of simulation does not provide the professional and social nature of actual IV insertion and therapy performed on a real patient. However, impact and fidelity are increased when students move from a task trainer to a created environment that authentically represents a practice environment complete with a patient, other clinicians, and variables of nursing practice (Figure 6.4).

Complements and Pitfalls

Traditional e-learning is didactic and focused on content delivery through either text-based or media content delivered via a course management system. In these cases, games, simulations, or virtual environments can be used to complement learning by providing the opportunity for students to learn by doing as opposed to being told what they *should* do (Aleckson & Ralston-Berg, 2011).

For example, when studying clinic management, information about key roles, duties, tasks, and management models can be delivered through text, recorded lecture, or other online media presentation using traditional e-learning means. After initial instruction occurs, learning can be enhanced in a virtual clinic. Encounters in the virtual clinic allow students to practice their management skills in an authentic environment that represents the variables and objectives discussed in during traditional didactic lessons.

This multiple approach process helps students gain experience in decision making, problem solving, group communication, and leadership. The objectives of the simulation taking place in the virtual clinic are in line with and map to the objectives of the instructional unit—to understand key management functions and implement them effectively under the environmental stressors of real-life professional nursing practice. The use of the added technology, in this case a simulation within a virtual environment, is relevant and provides instructional value to students. There is a measurable instructional return on investment to justify the time and resources spent to create, orient, and deliver the simulation.

In a contrasting example, the same clinic management unit could include a game that allows students to navigate through exam rooms within the clinic, gather clues from patients and staff, and locate some sort of treasure or reward within the clinic. Students may also need to blast "germ beasties" inside the clinic to clear the paths to the rewards and advance the game. In this example, learners may find the game fun and gather some peripheral knowledge about communication, problem solving, and strategy from playing the game. However, in this example activities represented in game play do not necessarily map to the specific learning objectives of the instructional unit. In this case the instructional return on investment would be too low to justify the time and resources necessary to develop it. As we discussed and continue to emphasize throughout this text, learning objectives and desired outcomes are the key to designing effective, efficient, and appealing instruction. To be sure a game, simulation, or virtual environment will complement learning, rather than create obstacles or distractions to learning, ask the following questions:

- Do the key functions of the game, simulation, or virtual environment map to specific learning objectives within the course or unit?
- Does the game, simulation, or virtual environment illustrate, model, or allow students to practice key concepts and tasks presented in the course or unit?
- Will the skills and knowledge acquired be useful in the learner's real-life practice?

A lack of reasonable expectations can limit possibilities and create pitfalls to successful integrations of games, simulations, and virtual environments that enhance learning. It is common for novice e-learning practitioners to assume that the addition of some type of game, simulation, or virtual environment will automatically increase interactivity and learning. In reality, as we have discussed and emphasized throughout this text, the use of such enhancements must be deliberately planned and designed for learning to take place. Another misconception is that nurse educators can serve as content experts, designers, developers, and support staff when it comes to implementing games, simulations, and virtual environments. It is difficult if not impossible for any one person to fill all of these roles. Curriculum design and development and content expertise, as well as technical support represent distinct areas of knowledge. We argue for and support a team approach to design, development, and delivery of simulation and game-based enhanced activities.

There are also potential pitfalls related to orientation and preparation. We have emphasized the relationship between preparation and learner success here and in previous chapters. Students who are not adequately prepared to participate may not succeed or may spend unnecessary and unreasonable amounts of time learning the system through trial and error.

However, we must be careful not to spend too much time on orientation and preparation. There must be a balance between time spent on orientation and time spent in participation. Well-designed environments should be intuitive. For example, a class of students is required to participate in a simulation. The simulation requires them to download, install, and use a software package to analyze data provided by the instructor over a one-week period. Students are using a diverse combination of computers, operating systems, browsers, firewalls, and security parameters for the course. The instructor must talk with each student individually and try to refer most to the software website for help. Most students have difficulty downloading and installing the software—so much so that most spend about 80% of their time downloading and trouble-shooting the software before they are able to begin participation. They spend about 20% of their available time during the week on the simulation. In this case, the preparation time required for active participation in the lesson plan does not justify the participation time.

Although it would be possible to create tutorials and request support staff to help students with the software installation, an alternative simulation that requires less preparation but meets the same learning objectives would be more appropriate. Technical support is not the responsibility of the student. Complicated technology with inadequate support frustrates students. Frustrated students are likely to be less engaged with the course.

We have previously discussed efficiency as one aspect of implementing games, simulations, and virtual worlds. A common pitfall related to efficiency is underestimating the time, costs, and support needed to implement a game, simulation, or virtual environment. For those new to implementing this type of learning, a more iterative approach can help manage resources. A rapid prototyping approach allows for prototypes to be quickly created and evaluated. When paired with documentation of hours and tasks completed, these prototypes can provide insights into the time and resources used for the project. Informed decisions and adjustments can then be made to keep the project within time and budget (Aleckson & Ralston-Berg, 2011). This information also helps to inform estimates for future projects.

There is also an ethical aspect to games, simulations, and virtual environments that must be considered. Warren and Lin (2012) raise the question of ethics in using games, simulations, and virtual environments for learning. They argue that students participating in role-play or virtual environments should be afforded the same considerations and protections as students participating in research studies. They recommend we consider potential risks and raise similar questions to those asked by institutional review boards. For example, is the game, simulation, or virtual environment appropriate for all learners? In considering *all* learners, are students with disabilities able to process information and participate? What are the possible risks of participation? Will learners encounter any values, behaviors, or identity conflicts that will impact them in a negative way? Will any unintended consequences or harm come to learners? Does the designer have the necessary skills to achieve all this? Is it possible for games, simulations, and virtual environments to do unintended harm to learners? The above questions must be considered to minimize risk and maximize learning.

To avoid pitfalls related to implementation of games, simulations, and virtual environments ask the following questions:

- Is there a viable alternative that will meet the same learning objectives but require fewer resources?
- Is the proper team assembled to create and support the game, simulation, or virtual environment?
- Can learners easily navigate from the main course content to the enhanced activity and back again?
- Are sufficient orientation and instructions included with the enhanced activity to minimize distraction and frustration while maximizing learning?
- Is the time required to prepare for the activity reasonable when compared with the time of participation?
- Does participation put learners at risk or expose them to dangers in any way?
- May *all* learners fully participate?

SUMMARY

When deciding what constitutes good curricular fit between technology and a curriculum, effectiveness, efficiency, and appeal must be considered. In proper balance, these three indicators of quality can guide the selection of games, simulations, and virtual environments in nursing education. Effectiveness ensures the technology has a positive impact on learning. Efficiency makes the best use of available time and resources. Appeal maintains student engagement and motivation throughout the learning process. All together they maximize the potential of games, simulations, and virtual environments for teaching and learning. To make the use of technology relevant and meaningful to students, its use must be aligned with the learning objectives in the course and units of instruction it is meant to enhance.

REFERENCES

Aldrich, C. (2009a). *Learning online with games, simulations, and virtual worlds: Strategies for online instruction.* San Francisco: Jossey-Bass.

Aldrich, C. (2009b). Virtual worlds, simulations, and games for education: A unifying view. *Innovate 5*(5). Retrieved November 24, 2011 from http://www.innovateonline.info/index.php?view=article&id=727

Aleckson, J., & Ralston-Berg, P. (2011). *Micro-collaboration between eLearning designers and instructor experts.* Madison, WI: Atwood Publishing.

Allen, I. E., & Seaman, J. (2011). *Going the distance: Online education in the United States, 2011.* Babson Survey Research Group and Quahog Research Group, LLC. Babson Park, MA.

Bonk, C., & Zhang, K. (2008). *Empowering online learning.* San Francisco: Jossey-Bass.

Boulos, K. M. N., Hetherington, L., & Wheeler, S. (2007). Second Life: An overview of the potential of 3-D virtual worlds in medical and health education. *Health Information and Libraries Journal, 24,* 233–245.

Chodos, D., Stroulia, E., & King, S. (2011). Developing a virtual-world simulation. *In Proceedings of the 3rd workshop on Software engineering in health care* (SEHC '11). ACM, New York, NY, USA, 71–78.

Conklin, M. S. (2007, February). 101 Uses for second life in the college classroom. *Second Life Symposium at the Games, Learning, and Society Conference*, June 23–24, 2005. Madison, WI.

Daft, R. L., & Lengel, R. H. (1986). Organizational information requirements, media richness and structural design. *Management Science, 32*(5), 554–571.

Dillenbourg, P. (2000). Virtual learning environments. *EUN Conference 2000, Learning in the New Millennium: Building new Education Strategies for Schools, Workshop on Virtual Environments.*

Fanning, R. M., & Gaba, D. M. (2007). The role of debriefing in simulation-based learning. *Journal of the Society for Simulation in Healthcare, 2*(2), 115–125.

Fanning, R., & Gaba, D. (2009). Simulation-based learning as an educational tool. *In Anaesthesia Informatics* (459–579). New York: Springer.

Gaba, D. M. (2004). The future vision of simulation in healthcare. *Qual Saf Healthcare, 13*(1), i2–i10.

Garver, K. M., McGonigle, D., Mahan, W. L., & Bixler, B. (2011). *Integrating technology in nursing education: Tools for the knowledge era.* Toronto: Jones and Bartlett Publishers.

Iwasiw, C., Goldenberg, D., & Andrusyszyn, M-A. (2005). *Curriculum development in nursing education.* Toronto: Jones and Bartlett Publishers.

Januszewski, A., & Molenda, M. (2008). *Educational technology: A definition with commentary.* New York: Lawrence Erlbaum Associates.

Johnson, C., Vorderstrasse, A., & Shaw, R. (2009). Virtual worlds in health care higher education. *Journal of Virtual Worlds Research, 2*(2), 1–12.

Kolb, D. A., & Fry, R. (1975) Toward an applied theory of experiential learning. In Cooper, C. (Ed.), *Theories of Group Process*. London: John Wiley.

Kozma, R. B. (1994). Will media influence learning? Reframing the debate. *Educational Technology Research & Development, 42*(2), 7–19.

Malone, T. W., & Lepper, M. R. (1987). Making learning fun: A taxonomy of intrinsic motivations for learning. In Snow, R. E., & Farr, M. J. (Eds.), *Aptitude, Learning and Instruction Volume 3: Conative and Affective Process Analysis*. Englewood Cliffs, NJ: Erlbaum.

Mili, F., Barr, J., Harris, M., & Pittiglio, L. (2008). *Nursing training: 3D game with learning objectives*. Paper presented at the Advances in Computer-Human Interaction, 2008 First International Conference.

Montoya, M. M., Massey, A. P., & Lockwood, N. S. (2011). 3D Collaborative virtual environments: Exploring the link between collaborative behaviors and team performance. *Decision Sciences, 42*(2), 451–476.

Nehring, W., & Lashley, F. (2010). *High-fidelity patient simulation in nursing education*. Massachutses: Jones and Bartlet

Pastore, R. (2002). Elearning in education: An overview. *Society for Information Technology and Teacher Education International Conference (SITE), 1*, 275–276.

Raths, D. (2006). "Virtual Reality in the OR". *Training & Development, 60*(8), 36–40. Retrieved on Nov 23, 2011 from http://findarticles.com/p/articles/mi_m4467/is_200608/ai_n21397142/?tag=content;col1

Reigeluth, C. M., & Merrill, M. D. (1979). Classes of instructional variables. *Educational Technology, 29*(3), 5–24.

Wadley, G., Gibbs, M. R., & Ducheneaut, N. (2009). *You can be too rich: mediated communication in a virtual world*. Proceedings of the 21st Annual Conference of the Australian Computer-Human Interaction Special Interest Group: Design: Open 24/7, November 23–27, 2009, Melbourne, Australia.

Warren, S., & Lin, L. (2012). Ethical considerations for learning game, simulation, and virtual world design and development. In Yang, H. H., & Yuen, S. C. (Eds.), *Handbook of research on practices and outcomes in virtual worlds and environments: Volume I*. Hershey, PA: IGI Global.

Weston, C., McAlpine, L., & Bordonaro, T. (1995). A Model for understanding formative evaluation in instructional design. *Educational Technology Research and Development, 43*(3), 29–49.

Wolf, M. S., & Duffy, M. E. (1979). *Simulation/games: A teaching strategy for nursing education national league of nursing*. New York: National League for Nursing.

7

Striving for Cultural Competency by Leveraging Virtual Reality and Game-Based Learning

RENEE PYBURN AND ERIC B. BAUMAN

OVERVIEW

*H*ealthcare professionals recognize cultural competency as an essential and required skill. In an increasingly mobile world it is vitally important to find effective teaching methods through which clinicians can achieve cultural competency. This chapter will provide an overview of cultural competency and its importance in the healthcare setting.

REVIEW OF THE LITERATURE

We will also review basic concepts and current applications of virtual reality and game-based simulations that support cultural competency and explore the possibilities for using these concepts to assist nursing students and other learners. Finally, we suggest guidelines for adopting virtual reality and game-based learning for cultural competency training and for future research on this topic.

CULTURAL COMPETENCE

What Is Cultural Competence?

There are various definitions for cultural competence in the literature. An often accepted definition of cultural competence is a set of congruent behaviors and attitudes defined by policies that allows professionals to work effectively in cross–cultural situations (Cross, Bazron, Dennis, & Isaacs, 1989; Isaacs, 1991).

Why Cultural Competence Is Important for Healthcare Professionals

Increasing Diversity

In many western countries populations are becoming much more diverse. For example, in the United States between 2000 and 2010, all major race groups increased in size (Humes, Jones, & Ramirez, 2010). African Americans, Hispanics/Latinos, and Native Americans represent more than one-fourth of the U.S. population (Humes et al., 2010). In one zip code in Queens, New York, people from 125 nations are represented (*National Geographic*, "All the world comes to Queens," 1998). About one-third of the European population under 35 years of age has an immigrant background. For example, in one public school with about 200 children located in Hamburg, Germany, 50% of the children represent more than 15 nationalities and speak about 20 different home languages (Gogolin, 2002). In 2010, it was estimated that out of the total population of Australia (22.3 million people), 27% were born overseas (Australian Bureau of Statistics, 2010).

Cultural diversity encompasses both healthcare workers and the patient population. The U.S. nursing workforce is composed of approximately 17% racial and ethnic minorities (U.S. Department of Health & Human Services, 2010). There is a documented movement of healthcare professionals from one part of the world to another, including a unidirectional movement of nurses from developing countries to developed Western countries (Cutcliffe & Yarbrough, 2007). Significant numbers of nurses migrate from Eastern and African countries to the UK (Cutcliffe & Yarbrough, 2007). In 2006, more than 20,000 licensed practical or registered nurses working in Canada were educated abroad (Hoag, 2008).

Healthcare providers must learn to step outside of their own cultural boundaries in order to provide culturally sensitive care to increasingly diverse populations, and also learn to step outside of their own cultural boundaries in order to understand the patient's cultural frame of reference. Clinicians must be able to understand the patient's point of view as filtered by his or her cultural frame of reference. Populations made up of a variety of cultural backgrounds make cultural competency training more complex because clinicians must be able to function effectively in a wide variety of cultural contexts. We argue that those working in healthcare should master the general principles of cultural competency. Ideally, clinicians and others working in healthcare should have an understanding of the different types of cultures commonly encountered in the setting where they work.

Each person's background and personal characteristics influence the way he or she views and understands people from other cultures. The factors that influence a person's culture and self-identity, and thus influence their cultural competence, include race, ethnicity, religion, gender, sexual orientation, age, disability, and socio-economic status (Office of Minority Health—U.S. Department of Health and Human Services, 2002).

Improvement in Patient Care and Safety

Applying techniques of cultural competency to clinical care can benefit patients and improve care. In a broader context this can improve healthcare delivery by reducing disparities in health services and increasing detection of culture-specific diseases. Delivering cultural competence at the macro level addresses inequitable access to healthcare, improves patient safety, and enables the provision of patient-centered care. Patient-centered care ensures that patients' preferences and beliefs are taken into account and that they have access to, and understand the information they need to participate in their own care (Institute of Medicine, 2001).

Lack of culturally competent care can result in the patient or family misunderstanding treatment plans and cause harm to the patient. For example, a clinician's lack of cultural framing can result in misunderstandings that lead to a patient not taking medication correctly, missing follow-up appointments, and poor adherence to treatment plans in the home setting. Thus, the healthcare provider must be able to communicate treatment plans effectively to patients with differing or limited language proficiency and diverse cultural backgrounds by providing culturally and linguistically appropriate services (Office of Minority Health—U.S. Department of Health and Human Services, 2002).

Requirements by Regulatory Bodies and Accrediting Bodies

Policies, laws, professional association guidelines, and schools require students to demonstrate a number of technical and nontechnical competencies in order to progress through curricula and maintain licensure and clinical privileges. Cultural competence is a nontechnical skill that should be evaluated as a practice-related competency. In addition, numerous healthcare professional associations, including the American Nurses Association, American Association of Medical Colleges, and the American Medical Association have urged schools to include cross-cultural medicine and healthcare disparities in their basic educational programs (Gilbert, 2003).

Accrediting organizations are reforming policies to better support cultural competence. For example, in 2001, the Liaison Committee on Medical Education (LCME), the nationally recognized accrediting authority for medical education programs, issued higher standards for curricular material in cultural competence than previously required (Liaison Committee on Medical Education, 2001). Specifically, the LCME requirements specify that:

> The faculty and students must demonstrate an understanding of the manner in which people of diverse cultures and belief systems perceive health and illness and respond to various symptoms, diseases, and treatments.

All instruction should stress the need for students to be concerned with the total medical needs of their patients and the effects that social and cultural circumstances have on their health. To demonstrate compliance with this standard, schools should be able to document objectives relating to the development of skills in cultural competence, indicate where in the curriculum students are exposed to such material, and demonstrate the extent to which the objectives are being achieved.

—http://lcme.org/functions2011may.pdf

Accreditation organizations such as The Joint Commission (TJC) require healthcare professionals receive training in delivery of services to diverse populations. U.S. federal regulations dictate that healthcare organizations provide culturally appropriate care through Title VI of the Civil Rights Act of 1964, as well as Medicare and Medicaid accreditation standards for healthcare organizations, medical schools, policies, activities and resources of professional organizations, and consumer advocate and minority interest groups (Office of Minority Health—U.S. Department of Health and Human Services, 2002).

In response to disparities in health due to socio-economic status, environmental factors, ethnicity, and gender, the U.S. Department of Health and Human Services (DHHS) has launched a number of major initiatives to improve the health of minority populations. For example, one of the overarching goals of the DHHS Healthy People 2020 project is to achieve health equity, eliminate disparities, and improve the health of all groups (U.S. Department of Health & Human Services, 2011).

Some population groups in the United States suffer disproportionately from poor health, disease, and limited access to healthcare. A study of the variance in healthcare among these groups culminated in an Institute of Medicine study and review document, *Unequal Treatment: Confronting Racial and Ethnic Disparities in Health Care* (Institute of Medicine, 2003). Several recommendations in this study begin to address and resolve these health and access disparities. One of these recommendations included the integration of "... cross-cultural education into the training of all current and future health professionals" (Gilbert, 2003, p. vi).

Cost Efficiency

Culturally competent healthcare contributes to better health outcomes and increased patient satisfaction. Cultural competency can also contribute to the provision of cost-efficient care (U.S. Department of Health & Human Services, 2001). It allows clinical providers to obtain specific and more complete information to make appropriate diagnoses. For example, when patient to clinician communication occurs in the patient's own language, cultural context is more likely to be understood as an integral part of the patient history. This in turn frames the immediate and future care of the patient. From this perspective, culturally competent healthcare plays an important role in the development of patient treatment plans. Culturally competent clinical staff are better prepared to attend to the unique needs of diverse populations and address cultural aspects of care at the level of individuals and their families.

Culturally competent treatment models reduce delays when seeking care, and facilitate and distribute health services more effectively among diverse populations. When patients perceive that clinicians provide care in a manner that respects cultural mores they are more likely to seek care in a timely manner. Further, patients can be reluctant to seek follow-up care when they perceive that during previous experiences clinicians did not provide care in a culturally appropriate manner. Simply making care available to diverse populations is something entirely different than having patients seek care and use available health services.

As discussed above, communication among clinicians and patients in the first or native language of the patient is preferable. However, it is unrealistic to expect that nursing and other clinical staff can consistently interact with patients in their first language. Miscommunication due to language barriers can have devastating clinical consequences. Facilities should provide appropriate translation services to enhance communication. Improved communication among healthcare providers and patients will frame the patient's cultural reference and healthcare beliefs and practices.

Seeing cultural competence as best practice enhances the compatibility between Western health practices and traditional cultural health practices. For example, some patients may prefer traditional healthcare practices or medications to Western models of care. Other patients may prefer a combination of traditional and Western healthcare practices. A culturally competent clinician should be able to elicit information about the patient and family's traditional beliefs and practices to find an appropriate balance between the traditional and Western methods of care.

Standards for Cultural Competency: National Standards for Culturally and Linguistically Appropriate Services in Healthcare (CLAS Standards)

The United States National Standards for Culturally and Linguistically Appropriate Services in Healthcare are commonly known as the CLAS Standards. There are 14 CLAS standards, first published in 2000 (U.S. Department of Health and Human Services). These serve as a guide for the provision of quality healthcare for diverse populations. Many healthcare organizations now follow these guidelines.

History of CLAS Standards Development

In 1999 the U.S. Department of Health and Human Services' (DHHS) Office of Minority Health (OMH) proposed national standards for culturally and linguistically appropriate services as a means to correct inequities that exist in the provision of healthcare in the United States. The OMH in the DHHS conducted a two-year study that resulted in the development of the CLAS Standards in response to the challenges associated with addressing diverse cultural practices found throughout an increasingly diverse U.S. population. One of these standards recommends that healthcare organizations offer staff education and training in the field for cultural competency (Office of Minority Health—U.S. Department of Health and Human Services, 2002).

The CLAS standards represent the first national standards in the United States for cultural competence in healthcare. The 14 standards comprise guidelines (standards 1–3 and 8–14) and mandates (standards 4–7) for all federally funded recipients. They follow three general themes: Culturally Competent Care (standards 1–3), Language Access Services (standards 4–7), and Organizational Supports (standards 8–14) (Office of Minority Health—U.S. Department of Health and Human Services, 2002). The CLAS standards are listed below (separated into the three categories outlined above):

Culturally Competent Care

1. Healthcare organizations should ensure that patients and consumers receive effective, understandable, and respectful care that is provided in a manner compatible with their cultural health beliefs and practices and preferred language.
2. Healthcare organizations should implement strategies to recruit, retain, and promote at all levels of the organization a diverse staff and leadership that are representative of the demographic characteristics of the service area.
3. Healthcare organizations should ensure that staff at all levels and across all disciplines receive ongoing education and training in culturally and linguistically appropriate service delivery.

Language Access Services

4. Healthcare organizations must offer and provide language assistance services, including bilingual staff and interpreter services, at no cost to each patient/consumer with limited English proficiency at all points of contact, in a timely manner during all hours of operation.
5. Healthcare organizations must provide to patients/consumers in their preferred language both verbal offers and written notices informing them of their right to receive language assistance services.
6. Healthcare organizations must assure the competence of language assistance provided to limited English-proficient patients/consumers by

interpreters and bilingual staff. Family and friends should not be used to provide interpretation services (except on request by the patient/consumer).

7. Healthcare organizations must make available easily understood patient-related materials and post signage in the languages of the commonly encountered groups and/or groups represented in the service area.

Organizational Supports

8. Healthcare organizations should develop, implement, and promote a written strategic plan that outlines clear goals, policies, operational plans, and management accountability/oversight mechanisms to provide culturally and linguistically appropriate services.

9. Healthcare organizations should conduct initial and ongoing organizational self-assessments of CLAS-related activities and are encouraged to integrate cultural and linguistic competence-related measures into their internal audits, performance improvement programs, patient satisfaction assessments, and outcomes-based evaluations.

10. Healthcare organizations should ensure that data on the individual patient's/consumer's race, ethnicity, and spoken and written language are collected in health records, integrated into the organization's management information systems, and periodically updated.

11. Healthcare organizations should maintain a current demographic, cultural, and epidemiological profile of the community as well as a needs assessment to accurately plan for and implement services that respond to the cultural and linguistic characteristics of the service area.

12. Healthcare organizations should develop participatory, collaborative partnerships with communities and use a variety of formal and informal mechanisms to facilitate community and patient/consumer involvement when designing and implementing CLAS-related activities.

13. Healthcare organizations should ensure that conflict and grievance resolution processes are culturally and linguistically sensitive and capable of identifying, preventing, and resolving cross-cultural conflicts or complaints by patients/consumers.

14. Healthcare organizations are encouraged to regularly make available to the public information about their progress and successful innovations in implementing the CLAS standards and to provide public notice in their communities about the availability of this information.

> —*U.S. Department of Health and Human Services,*
> *www.ombrc.gov/CLAS*

Achieving Cultural Competency

The goal of cultural competence training is mastery of specific knowledge and skills that increase healthcare professionals' ability to provide appropriate care to culturally diverse populations. This learning process should be ongoing and a part of all professionals' life-long learning process (Gilbert, 2003). Following are requirements for cultural competence within the health system:

Requirements for Cultural Competence within the Health System

- *Care* should be provided with an understanding of and respect for patients' health-related beliefs and cultural values and take into account disease prevalence and treatment outcomes specific to different populations. Care and treatment strategies should encourage and incorporate the active participation of community members and consumers.
- *Staff* should respect the health-related beliefs, interpersonal styles, and attitudes and behaviors of the individuals, families, and communities they serve.
- *Administrative, management, clinical, and organizational* assessment and processes should ensure a uniform and consistent response by all staff in every policy, procedure, and interaction.
- *Recruitment, retention, and training* of staff should reflect and respond to the values and demographics of the communities served.
      —*Requirements for Cultural Competence within the Health System: Primary Healthcare Section—Nova Scotia Department of Health, 2005*

The following are eight suggested steps provided for primary healthcare professions by the Nova Scotia Department of Health.

1. Examine your values, behaviors, beliefs, and assumptions.
2. Recognize racism and the institutions or behaviors that breed racism.

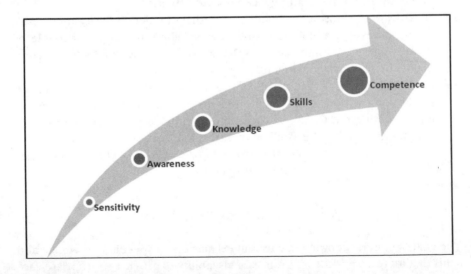

3. Engage in activities that help you to reframe your thinking, allowing you to hear and understand other worldviews and perspectives.
4. Familiarize yourself with core cultural elements of the communities you serve, including: physical and biological variations; concepts of time, space, and physical contact; styles and patterns of communication; physical and social expectations; social structures; mores; and gender roles.
5. Engage clients and patients to share how their reality is similar to, or different from, what you have learned about their core cultural elements. Unique experiences and histories will result in differences in behaviors, values, and needs.
6. Learn how different cultures define, name, and understand disease and treatment. Engage your clients to share with you how they define, name, and understand their ailments.
7. Develop a relationship of trust with clients and co-workers by interacting with openness, understanding, and a willingness to hear different perceptions.
8. Create a welcoming environment that reflects the diverse communities you serve.

> —*Primary Healthcare Section—Nova Scotia Department of Health, 2005, p. 6*

Cultural Competency Training Considerations

The goal of cultural competency training should be to improve the quality of care and provide enhanced service delivery to diverse patient populations. However, often the backgrounds of those teaching this content differ from the student population. Because trainers' backgrounds vary, the content delivered may be inconsistent. The person teaching lessons related to cultural competency will provide content based on their own cultural framing. That is, the teacher's own background and experiences influence how content is presented (Gilbert, 2003). This may result in inconsistency in the quality and content of curriculum and influence overall effectiveness of cultural training programs.

Those who have personal experience caring for patients from a particular culture or are from the same culture as patient populations being discussed may have a deeper understanding of the cultural framing and underpinnings of that culture. Instructors teaching within the context of their own cultural framing can provide authentic and expert experience to deliver more effective training about how to care for patients with similar cultural backgrounds. We argue that it is preferable to provide this sort of grounding because authentically situated instructors may be more effective in conveying cultural content than those instructors who lack personal experience with patients from such a background (Games & Bauman, 2011).

The focus of instructors who teach cultural competence training should center on the care-giving relationship between providers and patients.

It should also focus on how services are delivered to diverse patient populations. It is important that the content and knowledge base of different healthcare professions and how they are expected to interact with patients in a given clinical context is well understood. Those teaching cultural competence curricula should also have a clear understanding of the healthcare beliefs and practices among different populations to be served (Gilbert, 2003). Ideally, stakeholders from the community should be consulted and encouraged to assist in providing accurate information about that population's healthcare beliefs and practices, and general cultural identity.

Developing a receptive attitude on the part of educators, learners, and administrators toward cultural competence training is a critical first step to successfully integrating content into existing clinical curricula. Acquiring related skills, knowledge, and understandings specific to cultural competence follows (Gilbert, 2003).

It is important to provide nursing students with opportunities to practice culturally competent communication in order to help them develop relevant communication proficiency. Creating safe and appropriate environments where learning can occur is crucial. Simulation, specifically gaming and the use of virtual reality can provide learners with a safe environment to practice behavioral or non-technical skills related to clinical care prior to taking care of actual patients, particularly when addressing content that can be emotionally charged. Simulation and game-based teaching and learning can help healthcare providers learn more about the cultural context of the communities they serve, and communities learn more about how the healthcare delivery system works. This sort of collaboration will improve access to and quality of care through improved cultural competence (U.S. Department of Health and Human Services, 2001).

Guidelines for Teaching Cultural Competency

According to the "Teaching Cultural Competency" report (Office of Minority Health—U.S. Department of Health and Human Services, 2002) there are five guidelines to consider in teaching cultural competency (these are related to the CLAS standards):

1. *A patient-centered focus.* There should be a patient-based approach to cross-cultural curricula that focuses on differences between individual patients rather than between groups or cultures.
2. *Effective provider-patient communication.* Important concepts related to communication should include interviewing techniques and determining how best to explain treatment options and suggestions to the patient. This should include negotiation of treatment. For example, negotiation may include culturally acceptable treatment that combines Western-style healthcare with traditional health practices unique to the patient's culture.

3. *Balance fact-centered and attitude/skill-centered approaches to acquiring cultural competence.* Approaches to acquiring cultural competence should be fact-centered and attitude/skill-centered. The fact-centered approach to training enhances cultural competence by teaching clinicians cultural information about specific ethnic groups. However, a solely fact-centered approach may lead to misinterpretation that unfairly and inappropriately portrays patients as racial stereotypes. The attitude/skill-centered approach represents a universal approach to cultural competence that enhances communication skills and emphasizes the sociocultural context of individuals. Ideally, there should be a balance between the two approaches.

4. *Acquisition of cultural competence as a developmental process.* The acquisition of cultural competence is a developmental process. There are various examples of developmental models of cultural competence. Cultural competence focuses on methods and guidelines for practicing culturally competent care in multicultural situations. Acquiring cultural competence is a personal process of developing one's own cultural sensitivity and proficiency through self-reflection of one's own cultural identity and cultural beliefs. Experience with cross-cultural encounters are essential, and simulation in the form of gaming and virtual reality can provide such an opportunity for cross-cultural encounters (Office of Minority Health—U.S. Department of Health and Human Services, 2002).

5. *Understanding alternative sources of care.* Many of the conceptual frameworks regarding culturally competent care emphasize the importance for clinicians to recognize that patients may prefer and use alternative sources of healthcare and that their healthcare-seeking behavior is influenced by culture (Office of Minority Health—U.S. Department of Health and Human Services, 2002). That is, we must be aware that the contemporary Western healthcare system is only one alternative of many care delivery systems. Patients may turn to other resources including traditional beliefs and health practices rooted in diverse cultural mores to gain knowledge about and receive healthcare. Clinicians, including nurses should be able to provide strategy to reconcile contemporary Western models of care with patients' models, beliefs, and practices (Office of Minority Health—U.S. Department of Health and Human Services, 2002).

In summary, the achievement of cultural competency among healthcare professionals is widely considered an expectation for all care delivery. Including cultural competency training and demonstrating that it has been implemented among professional groups and healthcare organizations is often required by statute, administrative code, professional bodies, accrediting organizations, and clinical education programs. It is also a necessary component of safe, patient-centered, equitable, and quality patient care. What is not clear is the best method for providing this essential educational content and how to ensure that learners have achieved acceptable levels of cultural competency in a cost-efficient, engaging, and consistent manner.

Virtual Worlds and Virtual Patients

Virtual Worlds

Virtual worlds can be described as spaces that host synchronous digital environments that accommodate a persistent network of people, represented as avatars and facilitated by networked computers (Bell, 2008). There are training advantages of using an immersive learning environment like virtual worlds to teach facets of cultural competence to audiences of nursing and other clinical sciences students.

The distributed nature of digital environments is an advantage for cultural competency training. Virtual environments allow for virtual classrooms, virtual libraries, interactive role-playing, and remote seminars (Bauman & Games, 2011). Thus the need for an educator who is fully informed and qualified to teach others about a variety of cultures need not be physically present. When in-world experiences are carefully designed, the need for the instructor to be physically present may be reduced or eliminated (Bauman & Games, 2011; Games & Bauman, 2011). We can provide education in a virtual world environment where experts who are knowledgeable develop and write content about the particular culture or members of the culture being explored by students.

Students learning in virtual worlds have the advantage of access anytime and anywhere. They can also spend as much time as they desire immersed in training modules. This affords students the opportunity to glean experiences that may not otherwise be available in actual real-world clinical environments. In the United States it is possible for students to atttend and graduate from academic institutions with little or no contact with cultures different from their own. Digital worlds provide all students with opportunities for virtual first-contact scenarios to better prepare them for face-to-face clinical experiences. Virtual world experiences can provide learners with exposure to a wide variety of cultures and provide training opportunities that differ from traditional methods for providing cultural competency education.

Not only do virtual world or game-based teaching and learning platforms provide for student exposure to a wide variety of cultures, they also encourage students to take an active participatory role in their education. Providing experiences to adult students who support self-motivated learning and deliberate practice are consistent with *adragogy* (Merriam & Caffarella, 2007).

Educators can use immersive learning environments to model clinician-patient interaction, and clinical diagnostic skills (Bauman & Games, 2011). Thus nursing students and other clinicians can practice making diagnoses situated within various cultural contexts. Content related to disease processes, and wellness common in specific populations can be designed and presented in virtual worlds.

Other players can control virtual patients, or NPCs can be controlled by artificial intelligence, allowing students to have a natural language conversation with patients (Bauman & Games, 2011). Actual patient real-world conversations or situations (or adaptations of such) can be authentically re-created in digital environments. Virtual-world simulations enable students to practice professional behaviors in a risk-free environment (Danforth, Procter, Heller, Chen, & Johnson, 2009). This may be particularly important when the learner is inexperienced and exhibits anxiety about real-world encounters taking place in actual clinical settings with real patients. It also allows the learner to practice in an environment that eliminates risk of harm to actual patients.

Students receive virtual patients well. Their use as teaching tools improves cognitive and behavioral skills better than traditional methods (Dillon, Clyman, Clauser, & Margolis, 2002). Cognitive and behavioral skills are often difficult to teach effectively by traditional didactic and face-to-face teaching methods. Simply reading about and being tested on facts about cultural competence does not provide useful experiences to situate clinical encounters. Further, face-to-face role-playing exercises focusing on culture and diversity are difficult to facilitate in the absence of actual authentic cultural environments. In other words, it is not possible to replicate a clinical encounter authentically with a First Nations' patient without a First Nations' standardized patient. Attempting to do so risks creating an emotionally charged and unethical encounter based on stereotypes and cliché rather than expert and authentic practice. In the same vein it is unethical and ineffective for a Caucasian woman to play the role of an African American teenager.

Virtual worlds provide the opportunity for achieving learning outcomes specific to cultural competency training because patient–clinician encounters can be accurately, ethically, and authentically designed based on expert consultation and the actual lived experiences of the members of the cultures being represented (Bauman, 2011; Bauman & Games, 2011; Games & Bauman, 2011).

Participants can "step into the shoes" of practitioners or patients of different cultural backgrounds, and reflect on the consequences of their practice as a function of an overarching narrative. This is particularly important for cultural competency training. The malleability of game-based and virtual platforms allows for customization of cultural identity for characters in the virtual world. Creating situated environments based around the narrative of characters found in virtual settings provides an almost unlimited variety of possibilities to learn about different cultures. The combination of the activities, context, narrative, and characters represent the facets of culturally competent design. When these facets are thoughtfully represented in virtual spaces, the opportunity for rich and diverse cultural learning opportunities are limited only by the time and expertise needed to develop in-world cultural encounters situated for clinical education (Bauman, 2010; Bauman & Games, 2011; Games & Bauman, 2011).

Just-in-time and on-demand information can facilitate in-world problem-solving (Bauman & Games, 2011). For example, students review patients' charts prior to reporting to clinical rotations. Information in the chart commonly includes cultural information about patients. Innovative digital environments could allow students to leverage just-in-time virtual-world training just prior to seeing their real-world patients. These sorts of situated just-in-time learning encounters allow nursing and other types of clinical learners to engage in deliberate practice that specifically frames the real-world context of patient culture and ethnic identity.

Use of Virtual Worlds for Healthcare Education

The use of virtual worlds such as *Second Life* is increasing exponentially in clinical education. For example, *Second Life* has been used for disaster simulation, nursing training, and nutrition education (Danforth et al., 2009). A survey of the use of virtual patient simulation in U.S. and Canadian medical schools in 2007 found that 26 of 108 responding schools were producing virtual patients for clinical education. However, these virtual patients or avatars generally did not include patients with racial or ethnic diversity (Huang et al., 2009). The ability to create characters (both virtual patients and healthcare providers) in a virtual world with different cultural identities presents a golden opportunity to leverage the use of digital modalities like *Second Life* and game-based environments to help nursing students and other healthcare providers achieve cultural competency. The use of virtual worlds as a modality for healthcare education will continue to rise rapidly in the future, and the opportunity to take advantage of its flexibility and the ability to create widely diverse characters from a variety of cultures should not be missed. The variety of cultural backgrounds that can be represented is limited only by imagination. Educators can custom tailor characters from the backgrounds represented in a particular healthcare setting to match the learning needs of the nursing students and other learners.

Technical Aspects of Virtual World/Virtual Patient Design

It is important to give proper attention to the technical aspects of the design of virtual worlds and virtual patients (VPs) for cultural competency training. Among the factors to consider are flexibility, ease of use, scalability, portability, animation (fidelity to make the patient appear more human-like), linking facial expressions to the conversational output, and allowing for variations in the VP's emotional state that mimic real-life patients (Diener, Windsor, & Bodily, 2009). Flexibility in avatar design makes it possible to vary the cultural identity of patients and healthcare providers occupying the virtual environment. Flexibility or the ability to customize the created environment (Bauman, 2007) allows instructional designers to represent a variety of clinical settings. Ease of use, scalability, and portability of virtual worlds facilitate user-friendly applications for both faculty and learners. Improved animation to make the patient appear more human-like, linking facial expressions to conversational output, and allowing for variations in the VP's emotional state that mimic real-life patients improves the fidelity of the virtual environment and thus situates experience taking place in digital environments as authentic, immersive, engaging, and realistic for learners.

Leveraging programs that allow for optimal character or avatar customization is important. It is best to avoid ethnic, gender, and cultural stereotypes. Educators should base avatar creation on first-person knowledge of culture, or develop avatars through expert consultation. This said, we should balance decisions about the level of avatar realism with ability to drive psychological fidelity to attain suspension of disbelief of reality.

While software is improving to better model human movement and facial expressions, educational designers should take care to avoid the *uncanny valley* phenomenon (Mori, 1970). The uncanny valley is used to describe animated or robotic characters that approach human realism but lack fidelity specifically related to human emotion. The uncanny valley can evoke negative emotions and feelings among those viewing or interacting with these characters (Tinwell, Grimshaw, Abdel Nabi, & Williams, 2011). This phenomenon is illustrated by the animated movie *Polar Express* where animated characters were life-like, yet appeared vacant and emotionless.

Key Questions About the Use of a Virtual World as a Learning Environment

Diener et al. (2009) raise several key questions that should be asked about the use of the virtual world as a learning environment:

1. Is the virtual world sufficiently immersive for users to willingly suspend their disbelief in reality so that real learning occurs? Suspension of disbelief may be more effective if cultural competency training is based on actual patient encounters, diagnoses, and patient/provider conversations or patient histories and accurate and well-researched information about the particular culture(s) included in the training.
2. Some elements of simulations can be distractions. What level of abstraction might this apply to within a clinical simulation? How does this apply to cultural competency training?
3. What is the level of automated teaching that can be accomplished in simulations occurring in digital environments? Is the use of virtual worlds as learning spaces for cultural competency training most effective when used as a training modality in combination with other teaching methods rather than as a stand-alone modality?

Diener et al. (2009) uses both standardized patients and instructors to play the role of patients represented as avatars in real time in their *Second Life* virtual simulation center. Students and instructors are able to interact in the *Second Life* environment including various clinical devices and the virtual patients by using the heads-up display (HUD) or screen display. The University of Illinois–Chicago also uses a *Second Life* environment in a similar manner (Bauman, 2010).

The Use of Virtual Patients (VPs) for Cultural Competency Training

Virtual patients (VPs) represented in world as avatars are characters that are created using computer programs that simulate patients from real-life clinical scenarios. Learners can emulate the roles of healthcare providers related to situated tasks like obtaining a history, conducting a physical exam, and making diagnostic and therapeutic decisions (Games & Bauman, 2011).

Healthcare education has used VPs for a number of years for training undergraduate and post-graduate students as well as protective services professionals such as firefighters, police officers, and the military (Fors, Muntean, Botezatu, & Zary, 2009). In the United States Medical Licensing Examination (USLME) Step 3 in 1999 (Dillon et al., 2002), VPs were also introduced for assessment.

Universities develop most VP systems to reflect the needs of the institution in terms of the language, culture, procedures, and scope of cases (Fors et al., 2009). Given the costs associated with VP development, Fors et al. (2009) suggest universities and teaching intuitions should collaborate regionally and internationally. The European project, Electronic Virtual Patients (eVip, URL: www.virtualpatients.eu/, Retrieved May 26, 2012) is an example of multi-institution collaboration. Seven universities from six countries develop, share, and distribute VPs across cultural boundaries (Fors et al., 2009). These cases can be translated into multiple languages, and in some cases use language and quotation to form actual patients' clinical encounters.

VP cases that replicate actual patient experience provide a better approach to increasing the awareness and understanding of different aspects of healthcare. Basing the VPs and their cases on actual clinical encounters is more realistic and authentic than a "cookbook" approach. In other words learning by interacting with culturally diverse VPs provides a different and better experience than learning about culture by reading from a list of different cultural cues and characteristics (Fors et al., 2009). The following are examples of culturally related learning outcomes that could be targeted using VPs:

- Understand global health issues and possibilities/challenges in different parts of the world.
- Identify and reflect on personal cultural perspectives by encountering VPs with other cultural perspectives.

- Explore and understand the patient's different explanatory models and beliefs about health.
- Increase knowledge about cultural and spiritual issues through interaction with VPs to develop strategies for practice that attends to religious considerations and customs.
- Skills training regarding the management of cross-cultural interactions in patient care that promote trust and communication.

—Fors et al., 2009, p.737

Fors et al. (2009) also discuss the advantages of using virtual patients for cross-cultural training including the flexibility and adaptability of VPs as opposed to real patients where encounters are relatively arbitrary and non-negotiable. Fors et al. (2009) argue for the use of VPs to improve cultural competency by adapting VPs to different cultural aspects that promote learner understanding to identify strategies for coping with patients from different cultures, languages, social backgrounds, and medical conditions that students might encounter when caring for actual patients in the real world.

Holubar (2010) suggests that VPs existing in virtual worlds should be seen for a six month follow-up after the initial encounter. Doing so allows students to model the practice of continuity of care in virtual worlds that represents sound clinical practice existing in the real world. We argue that the development of virtual learning cases over time should be based on actual patient histories and cases. Since the virtual world is very malleable, learners can be given the option of developing and offering various care plans to VPs that include alternative therapies particular to the patient's cultural beliefs and healthcare practices, or a combination of Western and traditional healthcare practices. In this way multiple approaches to patient care encourage reflection about culturally competent practice.

General Considerations in the Use of VPs

- The selection and sequencing of cases to facilitate deliberate practice may matter more than the technical operations of the case itself
- The manner in which the feedback is provided and the ways in which the system supports the development of mental models may matter more than the fidelity of the simulated encounter
- When novices use a VP, they may have insufficient resources to construct robust mental models (cognitive overload), and thus may not be the best method for facilitating core knowledge development
- Deliberate practice may be facilitated by sequencing cases to ensure an ideal skill mix, structuring learning to develop constituent skills, and reinforce knowledge structures
- Provision of feedback, repetitive practice, progressive difficulty, and clinical variation

- Design of VPs probably varies for learners at different training levels
- Whether to make cases mandatory or optional
- How to integrate the use of VPs into the curriculum
- Whether to let students work in groups or alone
- Effective technological tools and savvy educators (experienced in using VPs effectively for learning) are needed
- How VPs should be used for assessment
- Technical support
- Ethical considerations
- Accessibility
- Usability concerns ownership of content
- Peer review
      —*Association of American Medical Colleges, 2007, p. 7; Games & Bauman, 2011*

Barriers to the Use of VPs

- Can result in inconsistent and limited use of VPs in clinical curriculum
- Requires complex programming and multimedia; time and resource-intensive to produce
- Confined within single institutions, resulting in potentially duplicative case development
- Successful integration and effective use hinges on the extent to which educators sufficiently consider curricular issues and training needs
- May require multiple funding sources
- Validating positive learning outcomes requires further research
- Barriers to sharing cases including:

  - "Not invented here" syndrome
  - Programs may be rigidly tailored to specific needs of a particular course or curriculum
  - Further refinement may require significant effort
  - Restrictive intellectual property policies
        —*Games & Bauman, 2011; Huang, Reynolds, & Candler, 2007*

Characteristics of the Use of VPs in Undergraduate Clinical Education:

- Generally used for individual learners rather than in small groups exercises
- Provides direct feedback to learners about their performance
- Peer review of case content is provided as part of curriculum development
- Tracking of user input and performance is captured
- Institutional intellectual property and learner activity is secure
- Most institutions are willing to share cases with academic institutions
        —*Association of American Medical Colleges, 2007*

Gaming: Cultural Competency Teaching and Learning

In the context of this chapter an educational game is a form of play, often competitive, played according to rules, and decided through skill (Allan, 1990). Educational or serious games are seen as a type of experiential learning. Learners engage in an activity, critically reflect on their experience, and extract useful insight from their analysis. This process situates the game experience so it can inform future professional and work-related processes (Pfeiffer & Jones, J.E., 1980).

The 2011 Horizon Report (Johnson, Smith, Willis, Levine, & Haywood, 2011) suggests that educational games can be broadly grouped into three categories. The categories include games that are not digital, games that are digital but that are not collaborative, and collaborative digital games. Games that are not digital and do not map well to digital environments are the sorts of games that require both face-to-face interaction and also include inherently haptic facets of game play. Numerous leadership development and strategy games requiring a physical group challenge fall into this category. Digital games that are not collaborative can be thought of as single-player games. Many computer or console-style video games are digital, but are not collaborative. In other words, the player is only interacting with the game, not other players sharing the same digital environments and experience. A good example of collaborative digital games is massively multiplayer online games (MMOGs). MMOGs exist in shared digital environments where collaboration and interaction with others in the environment is an inherent and intended part of game play.

Use of Gaming in a Transcultural Setting

While gaming as a teaching method is not new, using it to teach cultural competency is less common. In a study by Gary, Marrone, & Boyles et al. (1998) gaming was used in a transcultural setting as an educational tool in Saudi Arabia. In this setting nurses from more than 40 countries were represented from a variety of cultural, educational, and clinical backgrounds. The type of game used in this investigation was an adaptation of the television game *Jeopardy!*. The game was used to assist students who were engaging in distance learning to prepare for various examinations. The authors reported that using game-based learning in this setting helped the learners overcome ethnocentricity, communication barriers, language barriers, and cultural barriers such as the fear of "losing face" in front of peers by volunteering openly to answer questions that they might answer incorrectly. They also felt that this game-based learning intervention helped to promote critical thinking among cultures where outspoken and verbal autonomous critical decision making is not a familiar concept. By providing a nonthreatening learning environment students were comfortable and felt safe engaging in newly learned behaviors, such as enhanced communication and teamwork. Through various trials of the game the instructors learned how to improve their method of instruction. For example, teachers learned to avoid colloquial language and mannerisms. Further, teachers learned to distribute types of nationalities among groups rather than concentrating them in one group, and tried to be sensitive to player personalities in groups (Gary et al., 1998).

The type of game just discussed, a nondigital face-to-face activity, could be very advantageous as an educational method in a setting where there is complex diversity among staff in terms of both cultural and educational backgrounds. There are few studies exploring this concept, which highlights the need for further research to explore the use of gaming for the development of cultural competency. In summary, Gary et al. (1998) found that:

- Gaming can help overcome ethnocentricity and communication barriers, language, and cultural barriers among diverse groups of participants
- Gaming can help promote critical thinking skills, especially among cultures where critical thinking skills are not customarily valued or are unfamiliar
- Gaming can provide a non-threatening learning environment
- Gaming can provide learners the opportunity to demonstrate and apply acquired knowledge and skills, enhancing communication and teamwork
- Gaming can be fun for the learners

Although the example discussed previously included a game that was not digitally based, we believe that the same advantages can be realized using a video or digitally based game involving multiple participants or a first-person interactive game where a sole player interacts with multiple NPCs throughout game play. The cultural identities and other avatar characteristics (gender, age, educational background, personality type) of players in the game can be changed to provide cultural competency training for diverse populations. Varying avatar characteristics expose learners to a wide variety of cultural backgrounds and increases their experience and knowledge of different cultures. Placing learners in the "shoes" or "skin" of others teaches general principles of cultural competency. When students move outside of their own frame of reference they must try to understand and reconcile the frame of reference of a patient or colleague from a different cultural background.

Many of the advantages of using VPs and virtual worlds for teaching cultural competency discussed in this chapter and throughout the text also apply to interactive digital gaming:

- Flexibility and adaptability of the characters in games, as opposed to real patients where encounters are relatively arbitrary and non-negotiable
- Institutional collaboration and sharing of games can help reduce costs and time needed to create them
- Adapting characters within games to reflect different cultural aspects in order to allow learners to understand, and find strategies to cope with

patients with different cultures, languages, social backgrounds, and medical conditions than they might encounter with actual patients in real-world clinical settings

- Provide learners with an understanding of global health issues and the related possibilities/challenges found in different parts of the world by representing them in the game
- Learning to reflect on one's own cultural perspective by encountering characters with other cultural perspectives
- Exploring and understanding the "patient's" different models and beliefs about health and wellness
- Increasing knowledge about cultural and spiritual issues through characters that address spiritual issues and thereby allow for the reflection over strategies for religious considerations and customs (Post, Puchalski, & Larson, 2000)
- Developing skills training related to the management of cross-cultural communication
- Basing the cases and even wording used by the "patients" on real patient encounters/cases to increase realism for the student
- Game-based environments allow for the adaptation of the learning space to accurately reflect the learners' actual workplace
- The ability of online and web-based games to be accessed anywhere, anytime, and as frequently as desired by the learner
- The likelihood that game-based learning will be engaging for learners, especially those of the "Net Generation" or digital natives who enjoy and spend time playing video games (Prensky, 2001)

We realize that the scientific literature is limited as it relates to game-based learning in digital environments in general. It is scant at best within the realm of clinical education and cultural competency. We advocate for additional well-designed research that explores and validates the advantages of digital and game-based applications as an effective teaching method for cultural competency training. Further, it is important to explore how game-based and digital modalities can be effectively integrated with other teaching methods in order to achieve the best learning outcomes while engaging learners in a safe, nonthreatening environment.

Development of Video Games for Cultural Competency Training

Thompson et al. (2010) developed a nine-level action-adventure video game called *Escape from Diab*, targeted at 10- to 12-year-old children to educate them on how to better manage their diabetes. Through a series of focus groups, they found that youth preferred action games, an ethnically diverse cast of characters, physical attractiveness, characters that fit traditional gender roles, different levels of game play, and intellectual challenges. Engaging players in focus groups can evaluate this sort of player preference. Focus groups are a useful tool for developing any game-based intervention and should be used when developing games for cultural competency training (Thompson et al., 2010). Focus groups can be used to determine the preferences of the targeted learner groups. Games being developed should account for these preferences. Thompson et al. (2010) also found that goal-setting, problem-solving, motivational statements, goal review, feedback, and conducting debriefing sessions following game play may be helpful in facilitating learning through the use of video games. Incorporating these characteristics into serious video games used for cultural competency training may also be beneficial.

Criteria for Selecting Games for Cultural Competency

Sealover & Henderson (2005) suggests several criteria for selecting a game for integration into curricula and lesson plans. Among the criteria suggested are real-world relevance, flexibility (to allow for easy modification), cost-effectiveness, and user-friendliness. The same criteria also apply to the development of games for cultural competency training. Real-world relevance is an important facet of any situated learning experience. Relevance is important in the context of cultural competence game content and should be based on the cultural makeup of the specific patient populations or staff characteristics in the targeted settings. Content should attend to authentic dialog and health problems based on real patient encounters and histories.

Sealover & Henderson (2005) suggest that other criteria for selecting games should include appropriateness for predetermined learning objectives, participant involvement related to challenging tasks, and a scoring system that rewards achievement and makes learning obvious to the students. These characteristics relate to a successful gaming experience and apply across content including the selection of games for cultural competency training.

Considerations for the Proper Use of Games as a Teaching Strategy for Cultural Competency Training

Akl et al. (2010) list considerations for the use of gaming as a teaching strategy. These considerations include immediate feedback, decision making, not making the game overly complex, choosing the proper gaming format, and designing the game to meet learning objectives. These principles should also be followed when leveraging gaming for cultural competency education. Remember, elements and best practice for good gaming apply to all sorts of content. The point here is that gaming can be deployed for a number of educational concepts. Akl et al. (2010) advocate that any prerequisite knowledge that drives the intervention outcome be provided prior to the start of the game.

We have echoed this concept elsewhere in this text. Game-based learning is most effective when students are prepared for game play.

Guided self-reflection and debriefing are important aspects of any simulation or game-based learning program situated within clinical education. Debriefing is of paramount importance when using simulation and gaming to facilitate cultural competence curricula because the nature of the context and the lessons presented may be seen as emotionally charged and likely to address topics that make students uncomfortable. Self-reflection is an integral part of nursing and other types of clinical education. Encouraging students to reflect throughout game play, during active debriefing, and later to frame the context of new encounters is consistent with the various experiential pedagogies discussed throughout this text. Learning through and within digital environments compels students to negotiate their real-world identity with their in-world identity that culminates in the creation of the *projective identity* (Gee, 2003). The projective identity is discussed by Bauman in the context of nursing and more broadly clinical education:

> The *projective identity* emerges to represent learners' reflection on assumptions and implications associated with the reconciliation of their virtual and real-world identities. This reflection represents an essential opportunity to study aspects of cultural framing of self and other (Games & Bauman, 2011; Gee, 2003). Understanding cultural framing is important for nursing students because they are learning how to interact in new, different, and often uncomfortable contexts where culture and diversity can play important roles in physiological and psychological outcome (Schitai, 2004; Tervalon & Murray-Garcia, 1998; Thom et al., 2006). Further, cultural framing influences not only patient outcome but also facets of professional development and future work settings (Benner et al., 2009).
>
> *—Bauman, 2010*

Prensky (2001) states that games have 12 key aspects that are inherent to effective teaching. Some of these aspects seem particularly effective as a teaching strategy for cultural competency training. These aspects include the following: the element of fun, enjoyment, and pleasure; active involvement of the users; goals as motivators; ego gratification and personal satisfaction associated with winning; the benefits of competition/challenge; problem-solving interactivity; and emotional involvement. These characteristics make games fun and engaging. They should be seen as a strategy for cultural competency training and be incorporated as design elements in games specifically designed for cultural competency training. This said, it is important to understand that cultural competency is itself variable. Understanding cultural facets of one environment or population does not necessarily map to other contexts. We should design games so that we can modify them to be flexible and portable across cultural contexts and populations.

Assessing Learning Outcomes and Cultural Competency with Video Games

Built-in feedback tools and automatic scoring mechanisms can measure learner achievement related to cultural competency training within game-based learning environments. Attention to validity and reliability of assessment tools are important aspects of establishing and interpreting outcome. Validity and reliability may be both game and population specific. Learning outcomes can also be measured as a function of deliberate practice or time on task and total time of game play. Embedded assessment tools for the evaluation of cultural competency should include basic scoring of cognitive knowledge as well as more complex behavioral skill or nontechnical skills.

Rationale for Using Virtual Reality and Games to Teach Cultural Competence

Traditional Methods of Teaching Cultural Competence
Traditional methods for teaching cultural competence include classroom-based instruction, teaching at the bedside (with actual patients), the use of standardized patients (SPs), self-study, and instructor-guided case-based learning activities. Each of these methods has its limitations. The primary limitation associated with actual patient encounters and the use of SPs is that the variety of cultures that can be represented is left to chance. In other words, the type of actual patient the student happens to encounter during a given learning experience or the type of SP that is available limits the student's type of cultural encounter. Further, there are ethical and practical implications to take into consideration regarding using SPs to convey facets or variables of race and gender. There are limitations to the types of cultural differences that SPs can convincingly portray even when they are well trained.

Why educators should consider virtual reality and game-based learning for teaching cultural competency: Traditional methods of teaching cultural competency have limitations, and there are few if any methods to measure the comparative effectiveness of the various teaching modalities for achieving desired competency. We argue that game-based and virtual reality learning environments have potential as a pedagogical strategy for cultural training in nursing and other clinical disciplines. Additional research is needed to evaluate which teaching methods or combinations of methods are most effective for achieving the desired learning outcomes pertinent to cultural competence among pre-licensure students and nurses and clinicians seeking continuing education opportunities. Educators should consider virtual reality and game-based learning for teaching cultural competency because they provide the following:

- Potential for anytime, anywhere learning
- The ability to easily change the culture of the "patient" or "provider"
- The potential to use expert modeling
- The ability to change the language and context
- The ability to adapt to diverse communities and cultural groups from both the patient and clinician perspective
- The ability to change the healthcare setting to include multiple clinical settings such as the operating room, clinic, home, inpatient ward, or emergency department
- Cost effectiveness (once developed, can be used multiple times and across institutions)
- Sustainability
- Consistency in delivery of training
- The ability for learners to engage in an interactive environment
- The ability to practice first in a safe, non-threatening, non-patient care environment
- They can be partially integrated into multiple modes of content delivery
- They can vary case studies with endless possibilities
- They can build standardized assessment tools built into training modules that can evaluate the impact of training
- The training can give immediate feedback to the learner
- Ability to deliver unexpected events and unknown situations (Didderen, Wijngaarden, & Kobes, 2009)
- Student can learn at his/her own pace (Didderen et al., 2009)
- This modality appeals to today's "Net generation" or digital native learners (Prensky, 2001)

Despite the potential advantages, however, there are possible barriers to digital and game-based learning environments. These include the following:

- They can be expensive to develop
- Experienced multimedia developers are needed for their development
- Teachers/clinicians cannot develop and adjust cases to fit their own specific educational needs—they need specialized assistance from developers (Zary & Fors, 2003)

A Road Map for Using Game-Based Learning and VR to Teach and Achieve Cultural Competency

In this chapter we examined the reasons why cultural competency is a key competency for today's healthcare professionals, reviewed standards and guidelines for cultural competency, outlined the process by which cultural

Use of standards guidelines	• Use the CLAS standards (the 3 categories) as a framework[8] along with other recognized standards and guidelines for the provision of culturally competent care
Use of best practices	• Use recommended best practices in the development of cultural competence, including the steps in development (for example, the recommendations from "Cultural Competence Works: Using Cultural Competence to Improve the Quality of Health Care for Diverse Populations and Add Value to Managed Care" (2001)
Community engagement and expert input	• Engage with the communities being served to identify needs, to mobilize or create community resources to address those needs, and to continually reassess and redesign service delivery based on expressed needs • Involve those who have expert knowledge about the different cultures that are being studied in the development of training modules. Include members of the community or expert consultants
Staff training	• Ensure professional and ongoing methods of training staff so that delivery of training is consistent and developed and delivered by well-trained educators
Curriculum development guidelines	• Follow guidelines and best practices for development of virtual worlds, VPs, and games • Involve developers who are technical experts in the fields of gaming and virtual reality as well as educators who are experts in cultural competency training so that the games and VR training are not only well-developed from an educational perspective, but also that technology is leveraged in the most optimal manner to achieve desired learning outcomes
Research	• Through well-designed research studies, collect and evaluate data to determine the effectiveness of the use of these two learning modalities for cultural competency training. • Through research, determine the optimal combination of the use of games and VPs/Virtual Worlds with other teaching modalities to achieve cultural competency

FIGURE 7.1
Road Map for Using Game-Based Learning and Virtual Reality to Achieve Cultural Competency

competency can be achieved, and identified how cultural competency training is currently being approached. We then examined simulation, virtual reality and game-based learning, and their potential as methods for cultural competency instruction. We also provided specific attention and a discussion about the general advantages and considerations for these modalities and how they can be applied to cultural competency training.

Figure 7.1 is a proposed road map for using game-based learning and VR to teach and achieve cultural competency. The illustration provides several key steps that educators and administrators can use as guides in the development of cultural competency training through the use of virtual reality and gaming.

CONCLUSION

Cultural competency is an essential skill required for all of today's healthcare providers. Cultural competency is becoming ever more important due to increasing diversity of both patients and healthcare staff. Further, many regulatory bodies, schools, accreditation standards, and professional associations now require cultural competency training and achievement benchmarks. The use of virtual reality and game-based learning technologies are becoming much more common in healthcare education as instructional staff and faculty begin to appreciate their effectiveness as teaching tools. Further, these innovative multimedia methods of instruction have broad appeal to today's generation of learners (Prensky, 2001) who are comfortable with interactive digital media and social styles of learning that can be accessed anywhere, anytime, and can provide immediate feedback. The use of game-based learning and virtual environments accommodate flexible characteristics that promote facets of culture and diversity, including, but not limited to, the ability to alter the cultural identities of virtual patients, virtual staff members, other player and nonplayer characters throughout the environment and during game-play.

While we advocate for using digital environments and game-based learning to teach and evaluate cultural competency among healthcare providers, we recognize that there is very little research currently in this area. We also recognize that further studies focused on game-learning strategies in the area of healthcare and cultural competency using higher methodological quality are needed (Akl et al., 2008) to advance the scientific literature and the field in general. French (French, 1980) and others (Akl et al., 2008) suggest that games may be most useful as a follow-up or adjunct to other teaching methods rather than a stand-alone teaching strategy. Research to determine the optimal combination of gaming and virtual reality with other traditional methods of instruction to achieve cultural competency should be studied. In addition, the study of cultural competency training and awareness must itself be attentive to gender differences among learners in terms of the games that are most effective for individual or within cohort learning (French, 1980).

We believe that game-based learning and digital environments provide flexible learning environments that often do not exist in actual real-world classrooms or clinical teaching sites. While we advocate for additional research related to game-based learning and cultural competence, we see integrating these environments into curricula as part of the contemporary design and research process. In other words, developing educational interventions using games creates opportunities for further study and validation of game-based pedagogies. Most importantly, the relationship between achieving cultural competency through these types of training opportunities in the virtual and game-based learning spaces and actual performance in the clinical setting and patient outcomes must be studied.

REFERENCES

Akl, E. A., Sackett, K., Pretorius, R., Erdley, S., Bhoopathi, P. S., & Mustafa, R. et al. (2008). Educational games for health professionals. *Cochrane Database Syst Rev* (1), CD006411.

Akl, E. A., Pretorius, R. W., Sackett, K., Erdley, W. S., Bloopathi, P. S., Alfarah, Z., & Schunemann, H. J. , (2010). The effect of educational games on medical students' learning outcomes: A systematic review. *BEME Guide No 14, 32*, 16–27.

Allen, R. E. (Ed.) (1990). *The concise Oxford dictionary.* Oxford: Clarendon Press.

All the world comes to Queens. (1998). *National Geographic, 194*(3), Preceeding 2.

Association of American Medical Colleges (AAMC). (2007). *Effective use of educational technology in medical education: Summary of the Report of the 2006 AAMC colloquium on educational technology.*

Australian Bureau of Statistics. (2010). *Migration Australia, 2009–10.* Retrieved November 25, 2011 from http://www.abs.gov.au/ausstats/abs@.nsf/Products/07307EB8DDA18A92CA2578B000119743?opendocument

Bauman, E. (2007). *High fidelity simulation in healthcare.* PhD dissertation, The University of Wisconsin—Madison, United States. Dissertations & Theses @ CIC Institutions database. (Publication no. AAT 3294196 ISBN: 9780549383109 ProQuest document ID: 1453230861)

Bauman, E. (2010). Virtual reality and game-based clinical education. In Gaberson, K. B., & Oermann, M. H. (Eds) *Clinical teaching strategies in nursing education* (3rd ed). New York, Springer Publishing Company.

Bauman, E., & Games, I. (2011). Contemporary theory for immersive worlds: Addressing engagement, culture, and diversity. In Cheney, A., & Sanders, R. (Eds.), *Teaching and learning in 3D immersive worlds: Pedagogical models and constructivist approaches*: IGI Global.

Bell, M. (2008). Toward a definition of virtual worlds. *Journal of Virtual Worlds Research, 1*(1), 1–5.

Cross, T., Bazron, B., Dennis, K., & Isaacs, M. (1989). *Towards a culturally competent system of care.* Washington, D.C.: Georgetown University Child Development Center, CASSP Technical Assistance Center.

Cutcliffe, J. R., & Yarbrough, S. (2007). Globalization, commodification and mass transplant of nurses: Part 1. *Br J Nurs, 16*(14), 876–880.

Danforth, D., Procter, M., Heller, R., Chen, R., & Johnson, M. (2009). Development of virtual patient simulations for medical education. *Journal of Virtual Worlds, 2*(2), 3–11.

Didderen, E., Wijngaarden, V., & Kobes, M. (2009). *Emergency team training in virtual reality. An evaluation of the design process and of the performances of NIFV-ADMS in training sessions.* Paper presented at the SimTecT, Adelaide, Australia.

Diener, S., Windsor, J., & Bodily, D. (2009). *Design and development of medical sim second life and open sim.* Paper presented at the EDUCAUSE Australasia Conference. Retrieved from http://www.caudit.edu.au/educauseaustralasia09/program/abstracts/monday/Scott-Diener.php

Dillon, G. F., Clyman, S. G., Clauser, B. E., & Margolis, M. J. (2002). The introduction of computer-based case simulations into the United States medical licensing examination. *Acad Med, 77*(10 Suppl), S94–S96.

Fors, U. G., Muntean, V., Botezatu, M., & Zary, N. (2009). Cross-cultural use and development of virtual patients. *Med Teach, 31*(8), 732–738.

French, P. (1980). Academic gaming in nurse education. *J Adv Nurs, 5*(6), 601–612.

Games, I., & Bauman, E. (2011) Virtual worlds: An environment for cultural sensitivity education in the health sciences. *International Journal of Web Based Communities*, 7(2), 189–205.

Gary, R., Marrone, S., & Boyles, C. (1998). The use of gaming strategies in a transcultural setting. *J Contin Educ Nurs*, 29(5), 221–227.

Gee, J. P. (2003). *What videogames have to teach us about learning and literacy.* New York, NY: Palgrave-McMillan.

Gilbert, J. E. (2003). *A manager's guide to cultural competence education for healthcare professionals.* Woodland Hills, CA: California Endowment.

Gogolin, I. (2002). Linguistic and cultural diversity in Europe: A challenge for educational research and practice. *European Educational Research Journal*, 1(1), 123–138.

Hoag, H. (2008). Canada increasingly reliant on foreign-trained health professionals. *CMAJ*, 178(3), 270–271.

Holubar, S. (2010). Surgical serious video games. *Bull Am Coll Surg*, 95(1), 67–68.

Huang, G. C., Newman, L. R., Schwartzstein, R. M., Clardy, P. F., Feller-Kopman, D., & Irish, J. T. et al. (2009). Procedural competence in internal medicine residents: Validity of a central venous catheter insertion assessment instrument. *Acad Med*, 84(8), 1127–1134.

Huang, G., Reynolds, R., & Candler, C. (2007). Virtual patient simulation at US and Canadian medical schools. *Acad Med*, 82(5), 446–451.

Humes, K., Jones, N., & Ramirez, R. (2010). *Overview of race and hispanic origin.* URL: Retrieved from US Census Bureau website: http://www.census.gov/prod/cen2010/briefs/c2010br-02.pdf.

Institute of Medicine. (2001). *Envisioning the national health care quality report.* Washington, DC: National Academy Press.

Institute of Medicine. (2003). *Unequal treatment: Confronting racial and ethnic disparities in health care* Washington, DC: National Academy Press.

Isaacs, M. B. M. (1991). *Towards a culturally competent system of care, Volume II, programs which utilize culturally competent principles.* Washington, D.C.: Georgetown University Child Development Center, CASSP Technical Assistance Center.

Johnson, L., Smith, R., Willis, H., Levine, A., & Haywood, K. (2011). *The Horizon Report.* Austin, Texas: The New Media Corporation.

Liaison Committee on Medical Education. (2001). *Liaison committee on medical education annual medical school questionnaires.* Washington, D.C.: Association of American Medical Colleges (AAMC).

Merriam, S. B., & Caffarella, R. S. (2007). *Learning in adulthood: A comprehensive guide* (3rd ed.). San Francisco, CA: Jossey-Bass.

Mori, M. (1970). The Uncanny valley. *Energy*, 7(4), 33–35.

Office of Minority Health—U.S. Department of Health and Human Services. (2002). *Teaching cultural competence in health care: A review of current concepts, policies and practices.* Washington, DC: American Institute for Research.

Pfeiffer, J. W., & Jones, J. E. (1980). *Structured experience kit: Users guide.* San Diego: University Associates.

Post, S. G., Puchalski, C. M., & Larson, D. B. (2000). Physicians and patient spirituality: professional boundaries, competency, and ethics. *Ann Intern Med*, 132(7), 578–583.

Prensky, M. (2001). Digital natives, digital immigrants. *On the Horizon, 9*(5), 1–6.

Primary Healthcare Section—Nova Scotia Department of Health. (2005). *A cultural competence guide for primary health care professionals in Nova Scotia*. Nova Scotia Department of Health: Halifax, Nova Scotia, Canada.

Schitai, A. (2004). Caring for Hispanic patients interactively: Simulations and practices for allied health professionals. *Journal for Nurses in Staff Development, 20*(1), 50–55.

Sealover, P., & Henderson, D. (2005). Scoring Rewards in Nursing Education With Games. *Nurse Educator, 30*, 247–250.

Services, U. S. D. o. H. a. H. (2001). *CULTURAL COMPETENCE WORKS: Using cultural competence to improve the quality of health care for diverse populations and add value to managed care arrangements*. Merrifield, VA: U.S. Department of Health and Human Resources.

Tervalon, M., & Murray-Garcia, J. (1998). Cultural humility versus cultural competence: a critical distinction in defining physician training outcomes in multicultural education. *Journal of Health Care for the Poor and Underserved. 9*(2), 117–124.

Thom, T., Haase, N., Rosamond, W., Howard, V. J., Rumsfeld, J., Manolio, T. et al. (2006). Heart disease and stroke statistics–2006 update: a report from the American Heart Association Statistics Committee and Stroke Statistics Subcommittee. *Circulation, 113*(6) e85–e151.

Thompson, D., Baranowski, T., Buday, R., Baranowski, J., Thompson, V., & Jago, R. et al. (2010). Serious video games for health how behavioral science guided the development of a serious video game. *Simul Gaming, 41*(4), 587–606.

Tinwell, A., Grimshaw, M., Abdel Nabi, D., & Williams, A. (2011). Facial expression of emotion and perception of the Uncanny valley in virtual characters. *Computers in Human Behavior, 27*(2), 741–749.

U.S. Department of Health & Human Services. (2001). *CULTURAL COMPETENCE WORKS: Using cultural competence to improve the quality of health care for diverse populations and add value to managed care arrangements*.

U.S. Department of Health & Human Services. (2010). *The egistered nurse population: Findings from the march 2008 national sample survey of registered nurses*: Health Resources and Services Administration—Health Professions.

U.S. Department of Health & Human Services. (2011). *Healthy people 2020*. Merrifield, VA: U.S. Department of Health and Human Resources.

U.S. Department of Health and Human Services. National Standards for Culturally and Linguistically Appropriate Services (CLAS) in Health Care. Office of Minority Health Resource Center. Retrieved September 15, 2011, from http://www.omhrc.gov/CLAS

Zary, N., & Fors, U. G. (2003). WASP—A generic web-based, interactive, patient simulation system. *Stud Health Technol Inform, 95*, 756–761.

III

Evaluation

8

Assessing and Evaluating Learning and Teaching Effectiveness: Games, Sims, and Starcraft 2

MATT GAYDOS AND ERIC B. BAUMAN

INTRODUCTION

*N*ursing education has been a forerunner in the use of nondigital games and simulation for learning. Educators have used games to increase student interest in nursing topics (Horsley, 2010), to teach concepts such as immunology, ethics (Metcalf & Yankou, 2003), and pediatric cardiovascular dysfunctions (Cowen & Tesh, 2002), and to improve student skills, such as the use of evidence-based practice (Mohide, Matthew-Maich, & Cross, 2006). Faculties have used mannikin-based scenarios to train students for various psychomotor and behavioral tasks (Bauman, Joffe, Liew, & Seider, 2009). As the trend to adopt games and simulation into formal and informal education continues, nursing education faces theoretical and practical challenges. Rather than simply "tacking-on" such technology to existing programs, faculty and administrators who embrace newly developed curricula and interventions must understand how to take full advantage of games' and simulation's affordances. Assessing the effectiveness of these new educational programs and the various ways that games and simulation-based interventions can be exemplified will ensure quality control relative to program objectives.

Additionally, national education initiatives in the United States such as *No Child Left Behind* and *Race to the Top* have shown that assessment can be the principal driver of school reform (Collins & Halverson, 2009). Similarly, education objectives established as practice standards are exemplified in program assessments thus making changes to assessment methods a potential leverage point for enacting widespread program pedagogies. Research on assessment in the context of new pedagogy including games and simulation is essential for program and policy development and enacting reform.

Contemporary work in assessment research can help administrators and educators move from educational objectives or goals to the development of reliable and valid assessments that gauge program quality and may improve student-learning outcomes by providing frameworks that guide assessment construction. When coupled with digital technologies and assessments traditionally used in nursing, these models have the potential to provide more robust and economical methods of assessment and feedback than current methods alone.

Commercial video games also suggest new methods for building assessment and learning communities and offer tools that could be adopted for nursing education. In particular, games with a strong competitive community and tournament systems (for example, *StarCraft 2, Street Fighter IV*) provide assessment and learning resources for players in and out of the game. The assessment resources found in commercial video games serve as useful models for developing new instructional systems in more formal education domains. These resources also provide an understanding of how games and their communities of players support learning and can be used to inform the design processes for nursing education programs.

The purpose of this chapter is to synthesize current work in game and simulation-based learning, assessment research, and current trends in nursing education and to highlight specific ways that new programs might benefit from collaboration in these three areas. This chapter reviews the assessment framework *evidence-centered design*, the game *Starcraft 2*, and assessments commonly used in nursing including standardized patients and the objective structured clinical evaluation (OSCE). This review suggests that current research in learning and assessment on games and simulation provides support for improving nursing education outcomes, as well as student and program assessments.

NURSING EDUCATION

Accredited nursing programs exist in a variety of academic institutions including technical colleges, schools, and universities. These programs, which range from associate and baccalaureate degrees to graduate and post-graduate level training, are accredited by one of two agencies: the National League for Nursing Accrediting Commission (NLNAC) and the Commission on Collegiate Nursing Education (CCNE). Examples of agencies that accredit specialty areas of advanced practice nursing include the Council of Accreditation of Nurse Anesthesia Educational Programs (COA) and the American College of Nurse-Midwives (ACNM).

The role of accrediting agencies is to provide best practice in the form of standards and expectations for curriculum development, implementation, and evaluation. Derived from professional practice expectations in a number of domains associated with nursing, these standards are meant to ensure a minimum level of quality throughout the profession of nursing. Accreditation is meant to assure the general public, perspective employers, and the educational community that nursing programs have and maintain clear, appropriate educational objectives based on professional consensus and accredited programs continually work to achieve these objectives (CCNE, 2009; NLNAC, 2008). Additionally, accreditation establishes a criterion standard that ensures that assessments used to gauge and prepare students for professional practice are not merely reliable, but valid with respect to the demands of the nursing profession.

Common methods for making accreditation standards operational include written exams for licensure and supervised clinical observations. While written exams offer relatively valid and reliable methods for gauging student knowledge, they provide little information about how well the student will perform when faced with the inherent ambiguity and contingency of real patients in authentic settings. Clinical observations on the other hand, have higher face validity than written exams but suffer from challenges associated with sampling subjectivity and objectivity. In other words, who assesses the student and what observations "count" for assessment matter significantly when making judgments of student ability. Institutions often combine aspects of written exams and clinical judgments to develop a portfolio of student performance that accounts for both cognitive and behavioral performance.

Faculty develop student assessments from an institution's accreditation plan, often exemplified in the form of a rubric, which is referenced by instructors whose task it is to judge whether student performance meets satisfactory levels during clinical encounters. Administrators base clinical evaluations on the observations of nursing faculty and instructors. This method of assessment relies on the assumption that nurses with master's degrees have the expertise necessary to assess learners based on accreditation guidelines and administrative code set by each state's nursing board, and that such assessments are accomplished with an adequate level of validity and reliability.

VALIDITY AND RELIABILITY OF STUDENT PERFORMANCE

To be clear, we are not implying that faculty and instructors are not capable of making well thought out assessments of behavioral skills taking place in simulation-based, and later actual clinical environments. Rather, we are highlighting the difficulty of generating objective and standardized assessments of student performance in clinical environments, a long-standing issue in nursing education (Ross et al. 1988). For example, Miller (1990) describes assessment of student performance in this context as "essentially a method that depends on clinical impressions rather than systematic accumulation of reliable information. .... Applied occasionally it may have great usefulness in formative evaluation, but it has distinct limitations for summative assessment." (p. S64).

Miller (1990) cites two techniques sometimes used to address the challenge of subjective clinical assessment: the practice of using a standardized patient (SP) to assess clinical competency and the objective structured clinical examination (OSCE). Standardized patients are people, sometimes other students who have been prepared to act as patients, used to assess the skills of healthcare students and provide useful feedback on their performance. They have been successfully used in nursing education, and evidence supports their increased efficacy versus traditional methods of clinical evaluation (M. S. Yoo & Yoo, 2003). SPs are simulation at their core and, as such, are one level removed from actual patient encounters. Nevertheless, they offer close approximations to reality and are particularly useful for clinical education.

The OSCE is another useful resource for clinical training that has been used for over 30 years, especially in the UK, for evaluating nursing students' clinical skills (Harden & Gleeson, 1979; Ward & Barrett, 2009). In a typical OSCE session, students complete a number of unique stations. At each, they might perform a clinical task, answer questions, or attend to a standardized patient, usually observed by a content expert who provides an assessment of student performance. After a predetermined amount of time, usually a few minutes, students rotate to a new station until all students have completed all stations. The structure of the OSCE encourages uniform sampling of student performance and ensures the same assessor across the group, both of which contribute to increased objectivity and reliability (Rushforth, 2007; Walsh, Bailey, & Koren, 2009).

However, shortcomings of the OSCE include the high costs (upward of hundreds of dollars per student per session) as well as the potential to reduce nursing to a set of skills and patients to a list of symptoms (Nicol & Freeth, 1998). Further, the psychometric properties of the OSCE must be explored in more depth to ensure a minimum level of quality for all of the permutations of OSCE that exist. Nevertheless, when educators accompany assessment drawn from the OSCE program by written exams and observations of students in authentic clinical practice, a picture of student performance can be considered relatively robust and has been lauded as a "gold standard" for student evaluation (Carraccio & Englander, 2000).

This combination of assessment tools used in nursing education programs provides, at least in theory, a thorough framework for assessing student skills and abilities before they graduate and enter the workforce. However, we argue that the task of assessing students, evaluating education program efficacy, and efficacy of student learning can be improved with the use of games and simulations and the application of the learning principles that they embody.

Specifically, games and simulation provide the following:

1. More detailed and timely information about student performance.
2. Create low-stakes environments where students can fail in order to improve.
3. Multilevel feedback to relevant education stakeholders, including the student, instructor/faculty, and institution.

Thus games and simulation offer the potential to increase student interest in nursing and related fields and to improve the overall quality of nursing education and professional development.

The remainder of this chapter outlines current educational theoretical perspectives on games and simulation related to assessment, briefly reviews relevant concepts in assessment theory, and introduces current examples of games-based assessments from commercial entertainment games that may be informative for developing nursing education programs.

GAMES AND SIMULATION AS EDUCATIONAL TOOLS

Why Use Games and Simulation?

Researchers regard video games and simulation as essential to the reform of a struggling U.S. education system (Gee, 2004; National Research Council, 2011; Shaffer, Squire, Halverson, & Gee, 2005). Alarmingly high dropout rates among high school students and relatively low scores on international standardized tests have stirred researchers, policy makers, and educators to call for widespread change, arguing that because the current system is outdated, it is inappropriately preparing students for employment and active participation in an informed democracy. As it exists today, the U.S. public education system prepares students for an industrial model of society based on a manufacturing-based economy rather than for a technology-rich and increasingly dynamic global market model (Collins & Halverson, 2009; Tyack, 1974). Though the school system is particularly good at creating students with stores of disciplined knowledge and getting many of them into college (albeit some more than others), it does little to prepare students to adapt to a job market that requires frequent retraining, collaboration, and technological savvy. Games and simulation, researchers argue, may help to address these challenges as games and simulation exemplify many contemporary learning theories and support communities of self-motivated learners. If lessons from these new technologies can be understood and applied to domains such as nursing, educational environments may better prepare students for diverse, quickly changing, and technology-rich work environments.

Specifically, supporters of using games and simulation for learning point out the cultural ubiquity of commercial video games and the growing body of empirical evidence supporting the use of games as learning tools (National Research Council, 2011). Anthropologists investigating the play habits of young people have found that video games are played by nearly all of American youths, with close to 99% of teens reporting that they play video games of some sort (Ito et al., 2009). Although video gamers were previously stereotyped as antisocial teenage males, new generations of gamers are increasingly diverse, crossing socioeconomic status and gender boundaries (Ito et al., 2009). Further, the Entertainment Software Association reports that the average age of game players sampled is 37 and that a greater proportion of game players are women over the age of 18 than are males under the age of 17 (ESA, 2011). Video games offer educators the opportunity for widespread impact and provide a new medium to connect to a diverse audience of students, including nontraditional returning adult learners. While Mayo (2009) proposes this argument specifically for using video games to engage students in science, technology, engineering, and mathematics, the argument readily applies to nursing and other health-related fields as well.

The ubiquity argument is further supported by findings from learning scientists and education experts that point out that commercial games often exemplify many contemporary learning theories (Gee, 2003). For example, as *designed experiences*, games teach their players through cycles of interaction with feedback and reward systems (Squire, 2006). Through these experiences, players come to learn to value certain actions and ways of performing these actions. Players develop strategies for success as they learn the boundaries and leverage points of the system supporting game play (Squire, 2006). In some games including massively multiplayer online games (MMOGs), the designed experience found within the game encourages players to construct and explore unique in-world identities that bridge real-world identity with in-game personas. For example, the narrative of the game might encourage players to assume the role of a scientist or soldier, healer, or warrior (Gee, 2003). In other games, like first-person shooters, the designed experience is such that a player must learn to quickly identify, attend to, and react to objects as they appear on screen. In-world player experiences like these have demonstrated significant improvement on visual attention and inferential reasoning tasks (S. Green, 2010; Green & Bavelier, 2003).

Good games compel many players to spend hours of time and effort to master game objectives. Many of these games are designed to explicitly support learning. This learning can occur at various levels, ranging from the perceptual, as in the case with action games, to the social, as in the case with MMOGs. Regardless of which learning theory one prefers, it is important to note that these studies provide converging evidence supporting games' potential for education.

When support for player assessment and achievement is not provided by the game itself, communities of players often develop their own tools to help overcome the challenges that are posed in each game and meet objectives of game play. Game communities are social spaces where players are afforded the opportunity to share their experiences of game play with others. Using websites and other online resources, players create Wikipedia articles to document and organize game information, and write detailed guides that describe how to beat a certain game. While the content that players are focused on in commercial game contexts are not often valued in the classroom, the skills that students acquire by learning to navigate these social spheres are valuable. In online discussion forums around MMOGs for example, some players engage in sophisticated and scientific forms of discourse and argumentation as they negotiate game meanings with other players (Steinkuehler & Duncan, 2008). Even while discussing the merits of elves or orcs, players learn to support their arguments with concrete evidence in order to make their case more compelling to their audience. The ability to develop and support arguments based on evidence is a critical and necessary skill needed to support nursing practice.

Further, game communities create spaces where players modify and redesign commercial games and share their new content with others. Through participation in these spaces, players can acquire skills related to game production and analysis as they transition from consumers to producers. By learning to modify and redesign their games, these players acquire experience with and knowledge of commercial quality design and technology (Squire & Giovanetto, 2008). Game communities allow players to engage others who are at various levels of expertise along the same content trajectory—similarly modifying, redesigning, or creating their own art in order to create new and often high-quality products. Some commercial developers have gone so far as to recognize this community development as a potential pipeline for new talent and have even hired new employees straight from these online communities. Integration of games into curricula moves beyond the discrete act of game play. The playing of games also provides learners with broad opportunity for learning that is related to the games being played.

Communities of gamers and player-producers found within these communities are interesting in the context of nursing education due to the way that they exemplify spaces where novices can observe and engage with experts, transitioning from consumer of knowledge to producer of knowledge. Developing virtual communities of nursing and other healthcare professionals that work directly with young people may increase student interest in related fields and may help students make the transition from being a recipient of healthcare, choosing careers in healthcare, and enrolling in nursing programs.

To summarize, commercial video games offer somewhat unique affordances that make them particularly good for education. That is, they:

1. Are ubiquitous among American youth.
2. Detail principles and theories of contemporary learning theory, including feedback mechanisms, opportunities for identity development, and social support structures.

3. Create communities that act as additional and equally powerful sites for learning (beyond the boundaries of the game itself).

As players interact with the game, share their gaming experiences with others, and participate in game-centered communities they learn discursive and technical skills that are valuable not only to members of the gaming community, but to society as well. Perhaps more importantly, formal education systems are struggling to retain students and adapt their pedagogies to contemporary needs and contemporary audiences. Games and simulation may help develop more efficient education systems that appeal to learners and prepare them for participation in a 21st century society and workforce.

GAMES AND SIMULATION BACKGROUND

In general, simulation and games are structurally similar. Both include rules or mechanisms that define how their components interact, require some input from the user, and imply the adoption of certain roles (for example, a pilot in a flight simulator). Simulation can be thought of as models that represent real or hypothesized phenomena in which users can manipulate parameters in order to observe outcomes (Clark et al. 2009). Unlike games, however, simulation does not necessarily encourage playful dispositions. Regardless, studies examining the effectiveness of simulation in classrooms have shown, similar to studies of games, that they can effectively improve learning. Educators have used games to teach chemistry (Stieff & Wilensky, 2003), physics (Jimoyiannis & Komis, 2001), electromagnetics (Iskander, 2002), geography (Carstensen, Schafer, Morrill, & Fox, 1993), and lake ecology (Ergazaki & Zogza, 2008). In nursing, SPs exemplify nondigital simulation. They are explicitly not playful and maintain certain structural elements of authentic clinical situations in which users, both students and instructors, are afforded the opportunity to see how certain inputs affect outputs based on pre-established rules.

Educators have successfully adopted games and simulation as education interventions in more formal education settings including classrooms as well as afterschool programs. Barab, Thomas, Dodge, Carteaux, & Tuzun (2005) researched and developed an online multiplayer virtual world called *Quest Atlantis*, which includes curriculum units ranging from water quality and lake science to writing and pro-social activities (Barab, Thomas, Dodge, Carteaux, & Tuzun, 2005). Squire, Barnett, Grant, & Higginbotham (2004), developed and researched a game that was successfully used to teach students conceptual understandings of electromagnetic physics. Clark, Nelson, Sengupta, & D'Angelo (2009) is currently working with a commercial educational game company to develop a physics unit focused on Newtonian mechanics. The theories and empirical studies put forward by these education researchers have provided games and simulation increasingly positive attention as potential candidates for providing education reform, even at the level of the U.S. presidential agenda (Gibbs, 2010).

The educational use of games and simulation is not without its challenges. These new media must overcome the same hurdles as their technology-based educational predecessors (Van Eck, 2006). In order for games and simulation to be used effectively as educational tools—especially in formal and informal learning environments—significant personnel, institution, and financial support are required. Games should not be considered a panacea to cure all of our educational maladies (Fletcher, 2011) and such systems will likely fail if the technology, rather than activity is expected to provide reform (Papert, 1987). Further, the relatively new educational games industry must learn how to produce, design, and develop the games that not only accommodate, but also take full advantage of the potential of the media. Each game project brings with it a unique set of learning objectives, assessment models, and implementation needs.

Nursing education faces many of the same challenges as other science-related domains. These challenges include:

- Raising interest and awareness about the profession, especially among minority populations (Childs, Jones, Nugent, & Cook, 2004; Taxis, 2006).
- Adjusting curriculum to contemporary issues such as increasing technology.
- Ensuring a minimum level of quality or standard of education across programs and subsequently quality of nursing students.

Current research suggests that games and simulation may be particularly adept at addressing the first two issues, as they are immensely popular and powerful learning tools. Similarly the affordances of games and simulation may provide potential for ensuring quality assurance across nursing programs while providing appropriate feedback to students and teachers. Though most current research programs have not focused on nursing education specifically, they provide evidence that games and simulation can be successfully used in formal education contexts, providing groundwork for developing programs in other disciplines. The following section introduces the literature on assessment in education contexts more broadly, and with games and simulation specifically.

ASSESSMENT AND LEARNING THEORY

The National Research Council's commissioned book titled *Knowing What Students Know* (2001) describes and characterizes assessment as a process of drawing inference from evidence. There are three elements that are essential to the assessment process: a set of observations of the student being assessed, beliefs or theory that explains what those observations mean, and a model or theory of student cognition. All assessments are contextual and should only be used to draw conclusions about student knowledge based in the context for which they were designed.

Further, in order for assessments to be valid, they should align with the intended outcomes of the intervention, predefined models of expertise, or some other external measure, such as a psychological construct. In his now canonical chapter on validity, Messick (1993) describes validation as a process of interpretive inference by which one "ascertains the degree to which multiple lines of evidence are consonant with the inference, while establishing that alternative inferences are less supported" (p. 13).

Assessments are neither inherently nor universally valid and an assessment's validity must be established through some external criterion. Validity can be considered in terms of the degree of the strength of the relationship between the evidence gathered and the inference or claim being made. For content validity, this relationship is based on a task or job analysis that examines forms of behavior among practitioners, paying particular attention to forms that separate "good" from "poor" performance (Messick, 1993). This criterion is the basis for validity, as it is not enough (though it is often more convenient) to validate by correlating measures with external assessments. Instead, validity must address the meaning of test scores via some theoretical or rational grounds. In the case of nursing, this often means connecting the assessments back to authentic professional standards, which in turn must be developed and agreed upon by professionals in the community of practice.

The theoretical grounds for validity that Messick draws from are rooted in epistemology. They are based on theories of what it means to "know." Though such theories are rarely discussed in journal articles that present the results of educational interventions, they nevertheless serve as the basis for assessment tools.

If one considers knowledge as evidenced by biological change, for example, neurological or direct observations of behaviors can serve as sufficient evidence when making claims that learning has or has not occurred. Learning, for researchers studying the attention benefits of action video games, is observed in terms of improved performance on certain tasks that require accurate, speeded responses. Rather than focus on the player's potential interpretations of the representations in such games, attention researchers are more interested in understanding how and why the speed at which an individual processes information changes as a result of play.

On the other hand, researchers who consider knowledge as inherently social and mediated by player attributes in addition to game representations study action and discourse in and around game environments. That knowledge, thought of as enacted or a process, suggests the need for different units of analyses that are more appropriate for measuring learning. These units of analyses, in turn, compose better or worse evidence for making claims about learning.

Views on learning dictate the nature of games-based research and, as a result, inform the development of reliable and valid assessments. It follows, then, that games designed to increase student knowledge of important nursing concepts like anatomy, communication, or patient assessment will look different from games designed to increase student interest in nursing as a career. Understandably, these interventions will also use different methods and metrics to evaluate their effectiveness.

Research on games and learning can be roughly generalized as stemming from two theoretical camps: cognitivists and socioculturalists. Both hold qualitatively different views on learning. Qualifying these perspectives allows us to more clearly define educational objectives that nursing education programs may wish to pursue, and subsequently the types of assessments (regardless of whether they are games or simulation-based) that are most appropriate.

COGNITIVISM AND SOCIOCULTURALISM

Many of the research programs examining the educational potential of games have done so from perspectives that draw on contemporary and often sociocultural theories of learning. Gee (2005) and Steinkuehler (2006) draw from the fields of sociolinguistics, situated theory, and embodied cognition in their discussion about the distinction between Game and games. To talk about the game (lowercase "g") means to discount what the player contributes to meaning-making within the game space and to treat cognition as predominantly residing in the head of the player. On the other hand, to talk about Game (capital "g") requires a consideration of the social, cultural, and political contexts in which the game is played and situates them as equally important in understanding the meaning that is constructed within the game space (Gee, 2005; Steinkuehler, 2006; DeVane & Squire, 2008). Games, they argue, should not be considered out of context, rather they must incorporate the relationship between the player, the game the communities with which the player is associated, and the social context in which the game is played. To sociocultural theorists, the context of play is not dissociable from learning that occurs. That is, in studying video games for their potential as educational systems, these theories point out that it is essential to take into account not only the game but the surrounding communities embracing the game as well.

Sociocultural perspectives are a relatively recent development; supplementing earlier work by cognitive scientists that characterized learning as a biologically based transfer of information (Anderson, 2005). Assessments in formal education settings today often subscribe to the biologically based transfer of information paradigm. For example, this type of paradigm would be interested in students acquiring an understanding of biological systems and would rely on theories of learning where the acquisition of specific knowledge and skills that support understanding of biological systems are considered the most important program objective. Unlike situated or sociocultural approaches, the cognitivist perspective frequently uses the metaphor of mind-as-computational device and considers the environment as influential but only a secondary factor that may influence learning or cognition. Cognitivism, currently the dominant paradigm especially in terms of student assessment, influences games and simulation studies by focusing researchers on measuring the knowledge, skills, and abilities of players.

This is an overgeneralization of both cognitivist and sociocultural perspectives as both consist of distinct variants and subvariants, of which many hold often-competing claims and assumptions. Nevertheless, to generalize these theories is helpful since the assumptions of cognitivism versus socioc700turalism have at least one substantial difference that, as we will see later, has pedagogical implications.

The cognitivist assumptions are roughly that the individual is considered the most important unit of analysis. What is of interest with regard to learning is what behaviors, skills, and knowledge are retained from one context to the next. Consider for example Wilson's (2002) summary of the embodied cognition perspective. Wilson (2002) explicitly argues that the environment should not be considered a part of the cognitive system due to its relative lack of stability over time and location (as opposed to the individual's mind and body). Researching the effects of the environment or the relationship between the individual and context is useful, but offers only supplementary information that may support or accompany studies that give primacy to the individual. This individual-centric notion is not new (Simon, 1996), but provides one difference between cognitivist and sociocultural approaches to knowledge and subsequently assessment.

That is, sociocultural perspectives, in contrast to cognitivist approaches, tend to consider the individual-in-context as an inseparable duality and the most important unit of analysis. To the sociocultural theorist (Lave, 1988; Lave & Wenger, 1991; Gee, 2002), learning is a product of the interaction between the individual and the material, social, and cultural environment.

Pedagogical implications can arise from the differences between these two perspectives. Socioeconomic factors play an important role in student performance. It would do students a disservice to exclude such factors from analyses and more importantly, fair assessment. Disassociating the individual from the environment when assessing performance and gain in knowledge may be unfair because of the influence of factors that are beyond one's control. For example, socioeconomic status (Dills, 2006) and the family structure prevalent in a student's school district (Caldas & Bankston III, 1999) are both significant predictors of student academic performance in schools. Considering this relationship it may be beneficial and more ethical to include assessments beyond those traditionally used in formal school contexts.

For example, programs that want to encourage student enrollment and interest in nursing careers might consider moving away from admissions standards based predominantly on traditional academic measures such as GPA, SAT, or ACT. New assessments and education programs rather, might consider introducing students to nursing programs in middle school or high school so as to assess student potential in context and provide education opportunities that are particular to nursing thereby raising student interest in the profession. Because nursing recognizes that standard paper exams are insufficient for a complete assessment, the profession may already be open to acceptance of contemporary approaches to learning that could lead to the development more reliable, valid, and inclusive assessments.

EVIDENCE-CENTERED DESIGN (ECD) AND STEALTH ASSESSMENT

Evidence-centered design (ECD) is an assessment framework that is currently being explored among some video game and learning researchers. According to ECD (Mislevy, Almond, & Lukas, 2006), assessment can be considered in terms of evidence-based argument construction. In order to make claims about an individual's knowledge, skills, or competencies, one must define and gather evidence used to support or prove some desirable claim. There are two major parts to ECD: a conceptual assessment framework (CAF) and the four-process delivery architecture. The conceptual assessment framework is comprised of the major elements of the assessment such as a probabilistic model of student knowledge as well as a model of the domain that is being tested. The four-process delivery architecture describes how the CAF operates in-context, for example determining what questions should be given to the assessee next or whether the test should be stopped entirely. For more on evidence-centered design, see Mislevy et al. (2006) and Mislevy, Steinberg, and Almond (2002).

To further clarify, consider the use of ECD in developing an assessment that determines whether a nursing student knows how to conduct a "standard" clinical examination. Even if it were possible to observe every student's assessment over the course of their clinical training, student knowledge cannot be directly observed. An approximation, or model of student knowledge is therefore assumed, and observable behavior is considered in terms of its relationship to this underlying model. This model is the *student model*. In order to relate observable behavior to the model, a set of rules is constructed. This rule set is the *evidence model*, according to which observations we make of student behaviors (evidence) are explicitly related to the student model. Experts determine what observations or evidence are important. Experts might inform us that there are basic elements that apply to nearly every type of patient assessment such as hand washing or using the patient pain rating scale. They might also inform us that there are more advanced elements, such as knowing and being able to state the indications and contraindications to administering epinephrine to treat patients suffering from anaphylaxis. Observing a student

washing one's hands appropriately and explicitly articulating when epinephrine should be used and when it should not be used can thus be considered
evidence.

The *assembly model* provides guidance for using the student, evidence,
and *task models* to accurately measure the desired domain. *The assembly
model* dictates the quantity and diversity of clinical conditions that should
be given to students when measuring general skills as opposed to more
advanced areas.

Finally, the *presentation model* determines the details of how the assessment will actually be administered. It might determine for example, that information will be presented in text or graphically, digitally or nondigitally, and
would document how nursing students might be asked to complete nursing
notes or care plans in relationship to specific aspects of assessment and
care delivery.

ECD can be used to guide the construction of a valid assessment device
in which evidence is used to support claims made about student knowledge
and skills, and it can do so regardless of the epistemological stance that one
holds. Researchers are beginning to use ECD in research about commercial
video games as well as game-like systems designed for educational purposes.

Shute (2011) applies ECD to commercial video games using what she
terms "stealth assessment" or assessment that is woven into the instructional
(typically digital virtual) environment. A stealth assessment system is comprised of a competency model, evidence model, and task model. The competency model is comprised of the knowledge or skills that are to be assessed.
The evidence model specifies the meaning of the collected observations,
describing the relationship between evidence and quantitative estimates of
learning. The task model specifies which tasks will be used to elicit observable
behaviors. Because stealth assessment draws on ECD, its core components are
essentially the same. What distinguishes the two is that stealth assessment
extends ECD into game environments, gathering data and making observations
of in-game player behavior. Stealth assessment illustrates the affordances and
challenges that are encountered when conducting educational video games
and simulation assessments.

Shute & Kim (2011) analyzed learning related to the commercial game
World of Goo, a game developed for entertainment rather than education purposes. In each level, players try to construct towers using the fewest pieces of
material possible in order to reach some in-level destination. In order to
develop their assessment framework, they first recruited experts for consultation and then conducted think-aloud protocols of players ranging from
novice to expert. Using the expert consultation and initial data from players,
they constructed competency, evidence, and action (renamed from task)
models, linking in-game actions to player competency. Four subjects were
used with this assessment model, and researchers scored players on in-game
proficiency as well as related categories (for example, problem solving and

causal reasoning). And though predictions of player achievement did not match whether a given player completed a game play level, Shute & Kim (2011) suggest that the player who scored higher on assessment measures was nevertheless, more learned than the player who scored lower. They conclude that:

- This highlights the importance of failure.
- Evidence-centered design can help researchers make claims about what it is that people are learning in commercial off-the-shelf games (as opposed to games designed explicitly for education and assessment) regardless of whether the game was intended for education initially.

ECD has also been applied to game-based educational systems (as opposed to commercial off-the-shelf video games) including epistemic network analysis (Rupp, Sweet, & Choi, 2010; Shaffer et al., 2009). Epistemic network analysis is based on a theory of epistemic frames, where learning can be thought of as the process in which individuals come to know the world, particularly with respect to a community of practice (Shaffer, 2006). According to this theory, knowledge can be thought of as "knowing with" or understanding how knowledge is related to the domain of interest, the identities of those within their community, their interests, and their associated practices (Shaffer, 2006).

In epistemic network analysis, student activities are considered in terms of a network of potential actions modeled after a professional practice. Student actions are tracked and recorded throughout an educational session and then related to the skill, knowledge, identity, values, or epistemology of the professional model. Results from early studies suggest that epistemic network analysis offers a new and potentially powerful method for tracking student learning as they play an epistemic game. Moreover, the method of analysis may be extended to other digital learning environments in which assessment is intended to take place via a situated theory of cognition.

DISCUSSION

Though the theoretical context of nursing education and learning in games or simulation (digital or nondigital) is similar, the needs of each with regard to learning outcomes, assessments, and audience are different. In general nursing education deals with very specific and discrete groups of students, such as undergraduate nursing students, graduate nurses just entering the field, or continuing/lifelong professional development programs tailored to continuing education. One of the primary goals of nursing programs is to ensure efficient and effective education that consistently produces high-quality nurses, where quality is defined by best practice in the profession.

Conversely, primary education deals with the general population regardless of student background or discrete student interest. Primary education operates with a different agenda and focuses on domain-specific learning related to general and accepted areas of learning comprised of an accepted curriculum where quality control (and subsequently assessment) focuses on preparing students to become informed participants in a democratic society (Dewey, 1916).

Sociocultural learning perspectives highlight the ability for games and simulation to create interest-driven and self-sustaining communities of learners that gradually move players from consumer to producers. Sociocultural perspectives of learning, particularly those that embrace game-based learning may increase student awareness and interest in nursing as a profession. Sociocultural models of learning provide a mechanism for moving students from a peripheral position where they are familiar with nursing and related concepts to a more central one that leads to careers in nursing.

THEORETICAL CASE STUDY: A SUITE OF GAMES

Consider a suite or series of games and simulations supporting nursing education.

Educators should design the games to meet different learning objectives and be used to incrementally increase student interest, awareness, and knowledge of nursing as the prospective student plays more of the games. The first game in the suite might focus predominantly on raising awareness of and interest in nursing as a profession by creating fun games and environments that highlight various aspects of the practice. This introductory game might focus on increasing interest in nursing among targeted audiences like middle school or high school students with the aim of sparking interest in healthcare fields.

A subsequent game in the series might be designed to convey specific concepts that prepare players for success in nursing school, covering for example, biology or anatomy especially as it relates to nursing. Such a game would shift toward representative simulation and could include specific didactic elements that would map back into the students' classroom activities in science courses. By providing content situated in nursing, such a game or simulation could facilitate positive emotions and perceptions about the field of nursing. This in turn might increase student interest in the type of academic achievement needed to gain admission to nursing programs.

One could imagine this suite of games and simulations being available as a progressive narrative beginning in middle school and high school, extending to college-level prenursing students and finally providing more advanced virtual clinical simulations to prepare students for actual clinical encounters. The culmination of this series might be designed to introduce and acculturate advanced learners to professional practice as they make the difficult transition from nursing student to practicing professional. This type of authentic and situated virtual simulation would focus on immersing students in scenarios that exhibit the contingency and uncertainty inherent to authentic clinical settings and expectations of the cohort they hope to join.

The games and simulation suite proposed here could be used to generate a community of learners similar to those that exist and are found in the commercial video game culture. Through this community, students could connect with peers and professionals in nursing, as such a space would afford visible and shared expertise among its members. Simulation and game-based learning environments and the patients they host exist in virtual environments that can be accessed online. This makes the kind of experiences outlined in this case study broadly accessible regardless of student location. In some scenarios simulated patients represented by avatars could be automated, allowing students to practice and routinize conceptual fundamentals independent of access to actual standardized patients or real-world clinical sites. Further, practice sessions completed in virtual spaces can be visible by experts and peers who could later offer constructive feedback and advice to improve students' knowledge, skills, and abilities. Though such a learning community seems idealistic and even unrealistic, it does provide a novel way to meet the growing need for education reform and for new nurses to meet the demands of an aging population and graying workforce.

ASSESSING THE STUDENT

Games and simulations with different educational goals would draw on different criteria for assessment. Basic-level games would likely leverage traditional measurement tools. For instance basic-level assessment might focus on determining whether students could identify anatomy or understood systemic relationships—both topics that students would eventually encounter in basic science courses and nursing school. Feedback in the form of in-game scores and classroom test grades should provide (a) players the opportunity for repeated game play for self-assessment of where improvements are most needed, (b) teachers the opportunity to address these areas of need, and (c) administrators with the ability to evaluate the program efficacy and determine the effectiveness of such programs in meeting established accreditation goals.

ASSESSING THE INSTRUCTORS

Teaching is a complex and difficult skill in its own right, and it is important to understand which instructors are more or less effective within formal education conditions. Understanding the way that instructors use games and simulation and characterizing good instruction when such tools are used may be helpful when teaching other instructors how to use such systems effectively. Similar to their students, instructors may have their participation in digital environments documented for review and sharing in order to reflect on what worked and what didn't within a learning scenario.

ASSESSING THE INTERVENTION

As institutions would likely need to determine cost-benefit tradeoffs of different educational interventions, assessment at the intervention level would look different than assessment at the student level. For example, where assessments for a nursing interest game could include interest surveys in order to determine if students' interest was increased, institutions could be more concerned with large-scale data sets that measure the effectiveness of the outreach and detail a model of the intervention. In addition to measures of interest, player demographics, game popularity, student grades, and enrollment trends might all be measured in the course of months or years in order to determine the successes or failures of a program. These measures are not unique to digital games and simulations and likely occur in some capacity already.

SUMMARY

Digital games and simulation provide evidence for assessment of student learning that sits somewhere amid paper-based assessments, mannikin-based simulations, and standardized patients. Digital simulations can be recorded in their entirety; student experiences within digital environments can be reviewed in greater detail than typically available during real-world clinical encounters. Faculty can monitor each action a player makes in the game environment for accuracy and timing. Teachers and students can review these sessions and, if appropriate, share them with others. This allows for collaborative feedback and constructive criticism. This is important not only from the perspective of the immediate lesson or objective, but also from the perspective of professional development.

Clinicians base the checks and balances of healthcare quality assurance on their ability to provide and receive constructive feedback to drive positive patient outcome. Distribution of student performance, among peers and faculty, represents a virtual "grand rounds" based on in-game performance and can support reflection on experiential learning. The ability to replay and document game and simulation experiences affords opportunities such as metacognition, which in turn can support deliberate practice skills improvement, and knowledge acquisition. Though these practices occur frequently in competitive activities such as sports and video games, education has yet to adopt and encourage similar activities. The following section on the commercial video game *Starcraft 2* provides a concrete example of how one competitive video game and its community carries out assessment on multiple levels.

Starcraft 2

Starcraft 2 is a real-time strategy game in which two or more players gather resources, construct buildings, research technology, and build armies that they then use to eliminate other players from the game. As a recent in-game news post states, "*Starcraft 2* is a lot of things, but at its heart it's a fierce strategy game rooted in fast-paced competitive play." It is immensely popular. It has sold over 4.5 million copies across five continents in 11 languages, and is currently one of the leading e-sports operating on a global scale. In South Korea, where the game is most popular, matches are viewed by live audiences and simultaneously broadcast to television stations and Internet viewers. Competitive leagues include sponsored players and organized teams that live together in houses in order to train together. The Global Starcraft II League (GSL) is currently in its 10th season and has awarded over 1.5 million USD in tournament winnings.

Professional games are regularly broadcast online and oftentimes include professional commentary or live discussions where viewers can talk directly to the player. Players competing online are ranked on a ladder system and scored similar to competitive chess or scrabble players.

In addition to being extremely popular, *Starcraft 2* offers interesting opportunities for assessment as its design and affiliations have helped to create an active and vibrant community of players where learning takes place via various means. The game provides an abundance of detail about each player's performance in each game. Game details include how many actions each player made, how many resources each player collected, how resources were allocated, and even what each player sees from their point of view or camera perspective. Players interested in developing new skills, such as which units to build and in what order, can get rapid feedback at the end of each game that can help them gauge whether they accomplished their goals, regardless of whether they won or lost. A graph of each player's army value over time is provided so that players can track their general economy and army growth over time. Feedback also allows players to see where encounters among their forces and other players armies took place.

Players can share previously played games through third-party websites so that players can solicit feedback of game play from more expert players or show off how well they played to their peers.

StarCraft 2 is a powerful learning tool due to the way that it exemplifies many learning theories based in both behavior and social science. Its user interface provides frequent and timely feedback, narrates game controls to provide new uses with instructions and strategies, and logs player actions for later review. In-game performance and assessment are difficult to disentangle because knowledge of the game and ability to play the game are observed rather measured via some external test.

Though massive amounts of knowledge obviously contribute to expert play, such knowledge must be combined and executed consistently against other expert players in order to gain recognition within the community of players who support *StarCraft 2*. Similar to nursing, performance in context is the gold standard for evaluating competency and expertise.

StarCraft 2 and supporting software also support learning by offering broad horizons of observation for players (Hutchins, 1995). Saved games can be replayed for allowing players to more easily diagnose areas for improvement. Frequently, games from advanced players are seen by hundreds of others around the world via live-streaming broadcasts. Amateur announcers have gained relative popularity by releasing prerecorded gaming sessions where they provide running commentary about the game play and cast interesting matches between players that viewers send them or that they create on their own. These casts provide newcomers with expert-level narratives of community games of various levels. Such widespread and approachable sharing is important for learning because, as Hutchins (1995) points out in the case of ship navigation, knowledge distribution within a community coupled with high visibility between novices and expert practice can help propagate learning.

In commercial video games as in other domains, repeated game play is not likely to be sufficient for improvement. Rather, cognitive psychology studies of expertise in domains ranging from violin performance to tennis show that deliberate practice is the best predictor of performance measures. Deliberate practice is even superior to games played and time on task (Ericsson, Krampe, & Tesch-Romer, 1993). *StarCraft 2* supports deliberate practice by providing data and feedback from games played.

Additionally, because games can be shared and are easily made public, individuals or communities of practice can be leveraged to help assess performance and make suggestions to the player/learner for improvement. Further, player performance data is also useful for game designers and publishers who are interested in making changes to their games as the community supporting the game evolves over time, in the same way that institutions are interested in the effects of educational interventions over time.

Blizzard, the company that created *StarCraft 2*, regularly updates the game to create better game experiences and adjust in-game elements to ensure that all changes are equitable for players. Because fairness or balance is difficult to gauge in the preproduction of game design, and can really only be accomplished once the game has been released, Blizzard uses player data to make game adjustments. Education programs can similarly use the rich data collection potential of digital games and simulations to adapt their programs to their educational goals to meet curriculum and student needs.

SUMMARY

Games and simulation may be able to address a number of nursing education needs. Games may be able to increase interest in the field of nursing among primary students and new college students. They may also provide prospective students with content that will better prepare them for success in nursing school and in the profession itself. Further, games and simulation could be developed to provide professional development opportunities for novice and expert nurses throughout their careers.

They also offer potential solutions to real issues currently facing the nursing profession, such as the growing need within the United States to attract students from minority backgrounds (Childs et al., 2004; Taxis, 2006) and the difficulty in creating veridical, didactic scenarios that can supplement clinical experience. Games and simulations offer new ways for students to experience elements of the profession in low-risk environments, provide educators with new methods for assessing student learning, and allow administrators to judge the effectiveness of educational interventions.

Creating valid and effective games and simulations in nursing contexts warrants continued research related to operationalizing and testing theories that have thus far been used predominantly in primary school settings. Continued research will provide an understanding of how research in other areas of general education applies to nursing education. Though novel pragmatic and logistical challenges will inevitably arise, nursing education already has a head start in using simulation for training and assessment, and thus has the opportunity to pioneer new lines of research for games and simulation education for itself and other health sciences.

Additionally, because nursing and primary school education share some similarities, nursing education can inform the fields of learning and assessment. Written standardized tests, for example, are often the primary way that students, teachers, and institutions are measured in public schools. To use only written tests is rightfully deemed inadequate for assessing nursing students and should be similarly considered inadequate for primary school students. That is, nursing education's successful use of simulation and clinical observations are parallel assessment tools that do not currently exist in public education or are infrequently used. Advances in the area of games and simulations in nursing education would likely be beneficial as research and theories developed for nursing that can then be extrapolated to other fields of research and practice.

REFERENCES

Anderson, J. R. (2005). *Cognitive psychology and its implications* (6th ed.). New York: Worth Publishers.

Barab, S., Thomas, M., Dodge, T., Carteaux, R., & Tuzun, H. (2005). Making learning fun: Quest Atlantis, a game without guns. *Educational Technology Research and Development, 53*(1), 86–107. doi:10.1007/BF02504859

Bauman, E., Joffe, A. M., Liew, E. C., & Seider, S. (2009). Simulation-based training to teach paramedics how to place and intubate through the use of LMA-FAstrachTM. *Simulation in Healthcare, 4*(4), 244.

Caldas, S. J., & Bankston, C. L., III (1999). Multilevel examination of student, school, and district-level effects on academic achievement. *The Journal of Educational Research, 93*(2), 91–100.

Carraccio, C., & Englander, R. (2000). The objective structured clinical examination. *Archives of Pediatric and Adolescent Medicine, 154,* 736–741.

Carstensen, L. W., Schafer, C. A., Morrill, R. W., & Fox, E. A. (1993). GeoSIM: A GIS-based simulation laboratory for introductory geography. *Journal of Geography, 93*(5), 217–222.

Childs, G., Jones, R., Nugent, K. E., & Cook, P. (2004). Retention of African-American students in baccalaureate nursing programs: Are we doing enough. *Journal of Professional Nursing, 20*(2), 129–133.

Clark, D., Nelson, B., D'Angelo, C., Slack, K., & Martinez-Garza, M. (2009). *SURGE: Integrating intuitive and formal understandings.* Poster presented at the DR-K12 PI Meeting, Washington D.C.

Clark, D. B., Nelson, B., Sengupta, P., & D'Angelo, C. M. (2009). *Rethinking science learning through digital games and simulations: Genres, examples, and evidence.* Paper commissioned for the National Research Council Workshop on Games and Simulations. Washington, D.C.

Collins, A., & Halverson, R. (2009). *Rethinking educaiton in the age of technology: The digital revolution and schooling in America.* New York, NY: Teachers College Press.

Commission on Collegiate Nursing Education (CCNE) (2009). *Standards for Accreditation of Baccalaureate and Graduate Degree Nursing Programs,* Washington DC.

Cowen, K. J., & Tesh, A. S. (2002). Effects of gaming on nursing students' knowledge of pediatric cardiovascular dysfunction. *Journal of Nursing Education, 41,* 507–509.

DeVane, B., & Squire, K. (2008). The meaning of race and violence in grand theft auto: San Andreas. *Games and Culture, 3*(3–4), 285, 264.

Dewey, J. (1916). *Democracy and education.* New York: Macmillan.

Dills, A. (2006). Trends in the relationship between socioeconomic status and academic achievement. *Social Science Research Network.* Retrieved from Available at http://ssrn.com/abstract=886110

Ergazaki, M., & Zogza, V. (2008). Exploring lake ecology in a computer-supported learning environment. *Computer-Supported Learning, 42*(2), 90–94.

Ericsson, K. A., Krampe, R. T., & Tesch-Romer, C. (1993). The role of deliberate practice in the acquisition of expert performance. *Psychological Review, 100*(3), 363–406.

ESA (2011) *Sales, demographic and usage data: Essential facts about the computer and video game industry.* Retrieved 12/2011 from (http://www.theesa.com/facts/pdfs/ESA_EF_2011.pdf).

Fletcher, J. D. (2011). Cost analysis in assessing games for learning. In S. Tobias, & J. D. Fletcher (Eds.), *Computer games, instruction.* Charlotte, NC: Information Age Publishing .

Gee, J. (2002). Learning in semiotic domains: A social and situated account, National Reading Conference Yearbook, *Vol. 51* (2002), 23–32.

Gee, J. (2003). *What video games have to teach us about learning and literacy.* New York, NY: Palgrave-McMillan.

Gee, J. (2004). *Situated language and learning: A critique of traditional schooling.* New York, NY: Routledge.

Gee, J. (2005). *Why video games are good for your soul: Pleasure and learning.* [Melbourne Vic.]: Common Ground Publishing.

Gibbs, R. (2010). President Obama to announce major expansion of "Educate to Innovate" campaign to improve science, technology, engineering and math (STEM) education. *Office of the Press Secretary.* Retrieved from http://www.whitehouse.gov/the-press-office/2010/09/16/president-obama-announce-major-expansion-educate-innovate-campaign-impro

Green, C. S., & Bavelier, D. (2003). Action video game modifies visual selective attention. *Nature, 423*(6939), 534, 537.

Green, S. (2010). Improved probabilistic inference as a general learning mechanism with action video games. *Current Biology, 23,* 1573–1579.

Harden, R. M., & Gleeson, F. A. (1979). Assessment of clinical competencies using an objective structured clinical examination (OSCE) In: ASME Medical Education Booklet No. 8. Dundee: ASME.

Horsley, T. (2010). Education theory and classroom games: Increasing knowledge and fun in the classroom. *Journal of Nursing Education, 49*(6), 363–364.

Hutchins, E. (1995). *Cognition in the wild.* Boston, MA: MIT Press.

Iskander, M. (2002). Technology-based electromagnetic education. *IEEE Transactions on Microwave Theory and Techniques, 50*(3), 1015–1020.

Ito, M., Bittanti, M., boyd, d., Cody, R., Herr, B., Horst, H. et al. (2009). *Hanging out, messing around, and geeking out: Kids living and learning with new media.* Boston: The MIT Press.

Jimoyiannis, A., & Komis, V. (2001). Computer simulations in physics teaching and learning: A case study on students' understanding of trajectory motion. *Computers and Education, 36*(2), 183–204.

Lave, J. (1988). *Cognition in practice: Mind, mathematics and culture in everyday life.* Cambridge, MA: Cambridge University Press..

Lave, J. & Wenger, E. (1991). *Situated learning: Legitimate peripheral participation.* New York, NY: Cambridge University Press.

Mayo, M. J. (2009). Video games: A route to large-scale STEM education. *Science, 323*(5910), 79–82.

Messick, S. (1993). Validity. In R. L. Linn (Ed.), *Educational measurement* (3rd ed., pp. 13–103). New York: MacMillan.

Metcalf, B., & Yankou, D. (2003). Using gaming to help nursing students understand ethics. *Journal of Nursing Education, 42*(5), 212–215.

Miller, G. (1990). The assessment of clinical skills/competence/performance. *Academic Medicine, 65*(9(suppl)), S63–S67.

Mislevy, R. J., Almond, R., & Lukas, J. (2006). *A brief introduction to evidence-centered design.* (Technical No. 632). The National Center for Research on Evaluation Standards and Student Testing: CRESST.

Mislevy, R. J., Steinberg, L. S., & Almond, R. G. (2002). On the roles of task model variables in assessment design. In S. Irvine, & P. Kyllonen (Eds.), *Generating items for cognitive tests: Theory and practice.* Hillsdale, NJ: Erlbaum.

Mohide, E., Matthew-Maich, N., & Cross, H. (2006). Use of electronic gaming to promote evidence-based practice in nursing education. *Journal of Nursing Education,* 45(9), 384.

National League of Nursing Accreditation Manual (NLNAC) (2008). National League of Nursing Accrediting Commission, Inc. Atlanta Georgia.

National Research Council. (2001). *Knowing what students know: The science and design of educational assessment.* Washington D.C.: National Academies Press.

National Research Council. (2011). *Learning science: Computer games, simulations and Education.* Washington D.C.: National Academies Press.

Nicol, M., & Freeth, D. (1998). Assessment of clinical skills: a new approach to an old problem. *Nurse Education Today, 18,* 601–609.

Papert, S. (1987). Computer Criticism vs. technocentric thinking. *Educational Researcher, 16*(1), 22–30.

Ross, M., Carroll, G., Knight, J., Chamberlain, M., Fothergill-Bourbonnais, F., & Linton, J. (1988). Using the OSCE to measure clinical skills performance in nursing. *Journal of Advanced Nursing, 13,* 45–56.

Rupp, A. A., Sweet, S. J., & Choi, Y. (2010). Modeling learning trajectories with epistemic network analysis: A simulation-based investigation of a novel analytic method for epistemic games, 319–320. Retrieved from http://epistemicgames.org/eg/wp-content/uploads/EDM-Submission-Rupp-et-al.-2010.pdf.

Rushforth, H. E. (2007). Objective structured clinical examination (OSCE): Review of the literature and implications for nursing education. *Nurse Education Today, 27,* 481–490.

Shaffer, D. W. (2006). Epistemic frames for epistemic games. *Computer Education, 46*(3), 223–234.

Shaffer, D. W., Hatfield, D., Svarovsky, G. N., Nash, P., Nulty, A., Bagley, E. et al. (2009). Epistemic network analysis: A prototype for 21st-century assessment of learning. *International Journal of Learning and Media, 1*(2), 33–53.

Shaffer, D. W., Squire, K., Halverson, R., & Gee, J. (2005). Video games and the future of learning. *Phi Delta Kappan, 87*(2), 111, 104.

Shute, V. J. (2011). Stealth assessment in computer-based games to support learning. In S. Tobias, & J. D. Fletcher (Eds.), *Computer games and instruction.* Charlotte, NC: Information Age Publishers.

Shute, V. J., & Kim, Y. J. (2011). Does playing the world of goo facilitate leraning? InD. Y. Dai (Ed.), *Design research on learning and thinking in educational settings: Enhancing intellectual growth and functioning.* New York: Routledge Books.

Simon, H. A. (1996). *The sciences of the artificial.* Boston, MA: The MIT Press.

Squire, K. (2006). From content to context: Videogames as designed experience. *Educational Researcher, 35*(8), 19–29.

Squire, K, Barnett, M., Grant, J., & Higginbotham, T. (2004). Electromagnetism super-charged!: learning physics with digital simulation games. *Proceedings of the 6th international conference on learning sciences*, ICLS '04 (pp. 513–520). International Society of the Learning Sciences. Retrieved from http://portal.acm.org/citation.cfm?id=1149126.1149189

Squire, K., & Giovanetto, L. (2008). The higher education of gaming. *E-Learning, 5*(1), 2–28.

Steinkuehler, C. (2006). *Why game (culture) studies now? Games and Culture, 1*(1), 97, 102.

Steinkuehler, C., & Duncan, S. (2008). Scientific habits of mind in virtual worlds. *Journal of Science Education and Technology, 17*(6), 530–543. doi:10.1007/s10956-008-9120-8

Stieff, M., & Wilensky, U. (2003). Connected chemistry—Incorporating interactive simulations into the chemistry classroom. *Journal of Science Education and Technology, 12*(3), 285–302.

Taxis, J. C. (2006). Fostering academic success of mexican americans in a BSN program: An educational imperative. *International Journal of Nursing Education Scholarship, 3*(1), 1–14.

Tyack, D. (1974). *The one best system: A history of American urban education*. Boston: Harvard University Press.

Van Eck, R. (2006). Digital game-based learning: It's not just the digital natives who are restless. *Educause Review, 41*(2), 16–30.

Walsh, M., Bailey, P. H., & Koren, I. (2009). Objective structured clinical evaluation of clinical competence: an integrative review. *Journal of Advanced Nursing, 65*(8), 1584–1595.

Ward, H., & Barratt, J. (2009). *Passing your advanced nursing OSCE: A guide to success in advanced clinical skills assessment: 1 (Masterpass)*. Radcliffe Publishing.

Wilson, M. (2002). Six views of embodied cognition. *Psychonomic Bulletin & Review, 9*(4), 625, 636.

Yoo, M. S., & Yoo, I. Y. (2003). The effectiveness of standardized patients as a teaching method for nursing fundamentals. *Journal of Nursing Education, 42*(10), 444–448.

9

Seeking Research Opportunities in Virtual and Game-Based Environments

ERIC B. BAUMAN, PAMELA KATO, AND MIGUEL LARA

OVERVIEW

Virtual and game-based environments present interesting and forward-thinking opportunities for educational research. Learning taking place in virtual and game-based environments meets and overcomes some of the challenges associated with distance, time, and fixed learning spaces for clinical educational purposes. This chapter emphasizes the importance of educational research when integrating new teaching methods into a course, curriculum, or across multiple curricula in an institution.

Further, this chapter discusses the challenges of evaluating the effectiveness of this evolving style of learning in clinically focused professions and the implications and impact over time. This discussion will provide examples of types of research and how they have been or could be included for education, organizational and patient safety objectives.

We address the role of the *Institutional Review Boards* (*IRB*) as it specifically relates to simulation and game-based research from an educational standpoint. Recommendations for communication with IRBs and IRB proposal preparation are also discussed. Our hope is to provide perils from the experienced to novices engaging in simulation and game-based research in large part because we advocate for and see research as an integral and necessary part of a clinical teaching institution's mission (Guy, Ratzki-Leewing, & Gwadry-Sridhar, 2011).

IMPORTANCE OF EDUCATIONAL RESEARCH

Research is vital to developing, integrating, and evaluating any curriculum. It is also important when making changes to a curriculum. Further, the process of maintaining a curriculum should be seen as an iterative continuous quality assurance process. Curriculum change is inevitable and occurs more rapidly in health sciences curricula than it does in many other fields of study found at colleges and universities. This occurs because technology facilitates scientific discovery, which in turn defines current and best practice. It is the educator's responsibility to ensure that what is being taught maps to current practice to ensure that pre-licensure students and students preparing for advanced practice roles are entering the clinical professions with the skill sets needed to meet professional practice expectations (Ben-Zur, Yagil, & Spitzer, 1999; Mawn & Reece, 2000). Consistent with healthcare's focus on evidence-based practice, curricula in the health sciences should similarly emphasize evidence as a basis for decision making.

Preparing learners for success revolves around three variables for the context discussed here. The first is content specific, or the "what" of the curriculum. It is established by curriculum committees at colleges and universities based in large part on credentialing and accreditation standards previously discussed in this text (CCNE, 2009). The second variable is "how" the content will be delivered. By "how," we mean how students will gain access to course and curriculum content. Traditionally, content delivery methods include lecture, small group discussion, and reading assignments. "Where" the content is delivered is the third variable. All of these variables have been discussed in previous chapters, specifically Chapters 1 (Bauman & Wolfenstein), 3 (Bauman & DeVance), 5 (Bauman & Wolfenstein), and 6 (Ralston-Berg & Lara). We have asked readers to be open minded about the "how" and "where" variables of nursing and clinical education. However, we have not discussed how these variables should be carefully considered and evaluated. Chapter 6 (Ralston-Berg & Lara) specifically focused on curricular fit when considering virtual reality and game-based learning tools for nursing and other types of clinical education. Here we stress the importance of evaluating technology like video games and virtual reality for their appropriateness for nursing and health sciences curricula prior to integration and further evaluating the impact of these learning tools on outcomes after integration into curricula.

The "how" and "where" of content delivery when engaging virtual reality modalities of teaching are explicitly connected, particularly when using the Internet for access to digital environments. New and novel learning spaces on the Internet and virtual worlds or gaming environments should be evaluated for efficacy. The current problem surrounding these new learning spaces and teaching tools is that much of the research evaluations to date have been poorly designed and carried out such that they are not suitable as evidence of efficacy (Akl et al., 2010; Kato, 2010). It is abundantly important that the investigations we conduct on these new learning spaces is conducted with high standards of research integrity (Kato, 2012a).

Evaluation of teaching environments pertains to digital spaces as well as to fixed space and in situ mannikin-based simulation. The questions to ask when evaluating environments as effective learning spaces can employ a qualitative or quantitative method of inquiry. The investigator should start with general research questions and move on to develop a specific hypothesis or hypotheses about said research questions. Research questions are developed based on a problem statement that is defined by the state of the current literature and the current practice environment. In this case, the state of games and simulation in clinical education (Akl et al., 2010; Marascuilo & Serlin, 1988; Polit & Hungler, 1999).

It is extremely important in any research endeavor to have a very good understanding of the academic literature in which you are conducting the research. This means you should know what the major findings are in your area and what kind of research has not been done. A clear understanding of what sort of research has been done will help to inform and establish your own program of research. Thoughtful and informed preparation will guide your research so that you can extend what is known about the research problem and contribute to the science of simulation and game-based teaching and learning in nursing and inter-professional education. For example, if the only thing known about the particular problem you are investigating has been revealed through studies that lack a control group, you can be assured you will be making a contribution to the literature if your research model includes a controlled trial. Proper and thoughtful preparation for your research will help progress your research finding and program to the "next step" or the "missing piece of the puzzle" that the journals will want to publish because it represents a contribution to knowledge and the scientific process.

Adequate preparation for research helps to inform you about the elements of previous studies you might want to draw from. Adequate preparation helps you identify measures from previous studies that have been shown to be sensitive in capturing changes in teaching tools that are similar to yours. For example, many video games have been developed with a theoretical basis in social cognitive theory (Bandura). Evaluations of these video games in randomized trials have shown that players demonstrate significant increases in their self-efficacy to engage in targeted behaviors compared to participants in control groups (Bandura, 2004; Brown et al., 1997; Kato, 2010). Thus, if you are interested in evaluating a new teaching tool that is driven by social cognitive theory, further investigation is of interest and warranted because previous research has consistently shown a significant effect on this variable. Engaging this research creates a win-win situation because (a) if you also find significant effects, your findings will be consistent with previous related research and provide evidence to support your new teaching tool, and (b) if you do NOT find effects or you demonstrate a negative effect, you have still found an interesting and unexpected finding. Either scenario contributes to the scientific knowledge and may be of interest to publishers and other researchers in the field of games and simulation. In general, spending the time to adequately prepare for research not only helps ensure that your research is relevant but it also gives you clues about which measures are sensitive enough to capture what is being impacted by your teaching tool.

Your background research will be informed by your research problem. The research question might be as simple as: Is a particular game-based environment appropriate to effectively deliver specific content associated with your curriculum? Based on the literature that exists on this problem, you can then formulate some specific testable hypotheses. The specific hypotheses related to your research question might include:

1. Students who learn through a game-based environment will demonstrate *greater* content knowledge acquisition as outlined in the course syllabus or approved school curriculum compared to students who learn in the school's traditional learning environment (lecture, traditional clinical settings, and small group discussion).
2. Students who learn through a game-based environment will *maintain* greater content knowledge over time as outlined in the course syllabus or approved school curriculum compared to students who learn in the school's traditional learning environment (lecture, traditional clinical settings, and small group discussion).
3. Students who learn through a game-based environment will *show improved human factors skills* compared to students who learn in the school's traditional learning environment (lecture, traditional clinical settings, and small group discussion) in their first year of postlicensure practice *based on blinded ratings of their performance in videotapes of standardized simulated clinical situations*.

As you can see, hypotheses can be broad or very specific. The formulation of research questions and hypotheses is often dependent on available resources and the objectives that the investigator hopes to address by completing a given research project.

Sample problem statement, research questions with corresponding hypotheses is provided below:

Sample Problem Statement

Simulation occurring in virtual or digital environments appears to be a viable teaching strategy for health sciences education. However, there is little empirical data indicating that in-world digital simulation is an effective pedagogical technique for health sciences education and evaluation (Nishisaki, Keren, & Nadkarni, 2007).

Research Question One

Does integrating a digital simulation in a virtual environment focusing on resuscitation training lead students to meet the cognitive objectives in an existing curriculum more effectively?

- *Hypothesis One*: Students will demonstrate greater increases in cardiac resuscitation knowledge from pretest to posttest as demonstrated by written examination compared to students trained with traditional didactic approaches including reading assignments, lecture small group discussion, and static mannikin-based resuscitation simulation.

Research Question Two

Are students who participated in the digital simulations in this course better prepared to manage crises than students trained through traditional approaches?

- *Hypotheses Two*: Students will demonstrate improved behavioral skills related to crisis resource management (leadership, followership, and communication skills) following the game-based teaching intervention, based on blinded behavioral ratings of subject performance captured on video, compared to students trained with traditional didactic approaches including reading assignments, lecture small group discussion, and static mannikin-based resuscitation simulation.

The researcher hopes to demonstrate in this example that the data demonstrate evidence of an increased cognitive and behavioral ability to manage a simulated cardiac resuscitation.

While this chapter does not provide a step-by-step how to process on how to conduct research on or in virtual and game-based environments, it is meant to help the reader identify opportunities for engaging in such research and the importance of engagement in research. It is imperative that teaching institutions evaluate their pedagogical practice. This means figuring out if your curriculum imparts knowledge to your students and more importantly in terms of clinical education, did students exhibit behavioral improvement from the educational experience that you offered them? Follow this process described in this chapter to evaluate both the curriculum and how you implemented it. Proper evaluation will use a good investigative or research process.

The current state of educational research related to games and simulations in clinical education is immature (Kato, 2010, 2012b; Randel, Morris, Wetzel, & Whitehill, 1992). Researchers should focus on studies that have robust research design and methodology to advance the evidence for effectiveness in this innovative field (Kato, 2012a). Poorly designed studies often lack internal and external validity (Schaefer et al., 2011).

Internal validity refers to how confidently the researcher can conclude that one can attribute the observed effect or outcome to the independent variable or intervention. In this sense the internal validity shows how confident we are that the outcome, a change of behavior or the acquisition of knowledge, is a result of the research intervention as opposed to some other variable (Cook & Campbell, 1979). Some common threats to internal validity in education research include difficulty of (a) blinding researchers and participants to study conditions, (b) implementing the teaching tools and control conditions consistently, (c) finding assessment tools that are not affected by fatigue or previous exposure to the assessment tool.

Researchers can minimize these threats by carefully reporting the details of the study and conditions that may lead to biases while standardizing study conditions as much as possible. In regard to standardizing conditions, one advantage of virtual and game-based teaching tools is that in many ways, they offer the researchers standardized teaching tools across a variety of environments. On the other hand, if researchers present the virtual environment or game as an explorable environment to encourage curiosity and learning, they may also lose control over their ability to standardize the parts of the environment to which participants are exposed. In other words, researchers may see explorable environments as engaging, but it is difficult to account for and control participant interaction within the environment. Fortunately, researchers can often track this information within the software for later analysis. However, they may find controlling for this variation can be tedious and of limited value if the study has inadequate power to detect these differences.

One of the best ways to minimize these effects and to improve the internal validity of a study is to evaluate a teaching tool in a true randomized experimental design. True randomized experimental designs are uncommon in educational research because they can be difficult to carry out. Studies using randomized experimental design are expensive and time consuming to conduct because they often require large samples of research subjects. Large sample sizes are often required to have adequate power to detect differences between groups. Despite this, randomized trials will always be considered the gold standard among quantitative research methods for demonstrating a cause and effect link between the teaching tool and the outcomes observed.

A randomized trial on a video game designed to improve medication adherence among young people with cancer by improving knowledge shows how helpful it is to include a control group when evaluating a game as a teaching tool (Kato, Cole, Bradlyn, & Pollock, 2008). Figure 9.1 is a graph of knowledge scores at baseline, one month, and three months for subjects randomly assigned to play *Re-Mission*, a cancer video game, or a control video game (*Indiana Jones*).

The figure shows that compared to the control group, the *Re-Mission* group showed significantly greater increases in knowledge about cancer compared to the control group. What is interesting is that the control group also

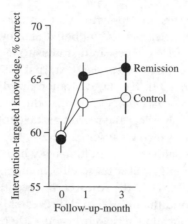

FIGURE 9.1

Differences in cancer-related knowledge from baseline to 1- and 3-month follow-ups in *Re-Mission* and control groups (From Kato et al., 2008, reprinted with permission from *Pediatrics*)

showed a significant increase in knowledge about cancer from baseline assessment. This suggests that merely the passage of time or, more likely, the act of taking a knowledge assessment repeatedly can lead to an increase in cancer-related knowledge. It has long been found that people tend to score significantly higher on exact or similar performance and achievement tests that they take the second time (Cane & Heim, 1950; Kulik, Kulik, & Bangert, 1984; Salthouse, Schroeder, & Ferrer, 2004). This effect was probably also taking place among the patients who played *Re-Mission*, but because their scores could be compared to the control groups, we could see that there still was educational value in this tool beyond these spurious effects unrelated to the learning game. However, if researchers did not include the control groups in the design, they would have misattributed the impressive increases in knowledge to the intervention itself. The control group actually allowed researchers to limit their claims to increases in knowledge beyond the effects of these "other" factors.

In summary, any research study that repeatedly administers knowledge assessment tools using a pre- and posttest design without a control group that shows improvements in knowledge is at risk for poor internal validity. The finding in the Kato et al. (2008) study emphasizes the critical role that control groups and randomized designs should play in evaluating teaching tools and improving internal validity of studies. In addition to using a control group, research studies can eliminate practice effects as a threat to internal validity by employing Solomon Four-Group design or a Post-Test only design (see Campbell & Stanley, 1963).

External validity refers to the extent that study findings can be generalized beyond the confines of the research study. In other words, do the research findings of a given investigation apply to other settings, teaching tools, evaluation measures, people, or learners (Campbell & Stanley, 1963)? Unfortunately, the more we tightly control our research studies to increase internal validity, the more we risk decreasing our studies' external validity. For example, the more participants we need to recruit to a randomized trial to have adequate power to detect differences between groups, the less likely it will be that we will be able to randomly select and recruit participants from that population because we need every available participant possible.

The more we standardize the conditions in which we evaluate our teaching tool, the less the findings will apply to environments in which the tool will be used in the real world. Thus the research intervention or tool may be less effective in the real world than it was in the research study. External validity is a key concern in education research because there is always a question whether research conducted in a controlled setting and manner will apply in the real world. Researchers can maximize external validity of research samples by random sampling of participants from research populations. Random sampling maximizes the possibility that the research sample is representative of the population to which it is intended to generalize. Once subjects have been recruited for any study, it may take significant effort to maintain the study sample. Measures such as compensation for the cost of participating in the study (travel expenses, time, etc.) and reminders about appointments may minimize the number of subject dropouts and missing data from the study (Cook & Campbell, 1979).

In the previous example discussing the *Re-Mission* video game, multiple knowledge assessments also represented a threat to the external validity of the findings because research participants may have shown increases in knowledge in both the treatment and control groups because they knew they were participating in a research study. Participants who are knowing and willing research subjects who expect to be evaluated and reevaluated a later point and may want to perform well and even excel during reevaluation. This is an example of the Hawthorne effect.

You will never be able to entirely eliminate all threats to external validity, however, there are strategies to minimize the threat. One strategy for reducing the threat to external validity is to conduct studies, collect data at multiple sites and settings that are more diverse and varied (Rothwell, 2005).

It is a daunting task to balance demands for internal and external validity in studies. One can take comfort in the fact that any research study is really seen as a bigger body of knowledge that provides converging evidence that either supports or fails to support a given theory. This goes back to the importance of doing background research. Those studies that have good internal and external validity offer the most significant contribution to converging evidence and understanding of the problem being addressed. This said, researchers must find a balance among internal and external validity particularly when conducting behavioral research with human subjects. By looking at the big picture found in the research literature, researchers can often find a balance to internal and external validity challenges.

QUALITATIVE AND QUANTITATIVE RESEARCH

This text does not take a stand on the appropriateness of qualitative versus quantitative research. The key point we stress is support for educational research that validates and supports the appropriate integration of games and simulations into health sciences curricula. Below are two brief descriptions of quantitative and qualitative research processes.

Qualitative Research Process

The qualitative research method attends to the following:

- Problem statement
- Purpose and research questions
- Hypotheses
- Literature review
- Framework or theory
- Methods section
- Results based on analysis
- Findings
- Discussion

The qualitative and quantitative methods, in principle, share similarities in process. However, the qualitative process takes a different approach to data and data analysis. With the qualitative approach we collect data through observation. This approach includes methods like interviews, focus groups, and analysis of text and documents. In general, researchers analyze data "as is" rather than as a statistical datum point (Polit & Hungler, 1999). Some examples of theories that motivate qualitative research and analyses include phenomenology, critical theory, and grounded theory (Diekelmann, 2003).

In terms of research planning, it is often very helpful to begin a research program with qualitative research. Qualitative research is a useful way to explore research problems and provides a basis for formulating specific research hypotheses that can be investigated by either further qualitative analysis or through a quantitative approach. It is helpful to start research programs with qualitative studies because researchers can often conduct them more quickly with fewer research participants and often more economically than with the quantitative research process. While some scholars subscribe and argue for an either-or approach in terms of quantitative or qualitative methodology, we argue that a sound research program can accommodate and leverage a mixed-method approach. Choosing a method should map back to the research objectives, or what one expects to achieve by completing the research. For example, findings from qualitative research studies may provide the basis for research grant proposals that fund and support quantitative research. This said, in some contexts qualitative research might stand on its own merits. Again, researcher objectives will determine which method is best suited for the goals and objectives of any given research program.

Quantitative Research Process

In general, the quantitative research process includes the following facets:

- Problem statement
- Purpose and research questions
- Hypothesis
- Literature review
- Framework or theory
- Methods section
- Results section based on statistical analysis of a numerical data set
- Findings
- Discussion section

Researchers often refer to or associate quantitative research processes with empirical studies and the scientific process (Polit & Hungler, 1999). Empirical studies and the scientific process are often a good basis for generating more specific hypotheses that we can test in rigorous research designs.

Engaging in research produces formative information to justify curriculum changes and encourage curriculum improvement. However, gaining proficiency and expertise in research is iterative. Novices should develop collaborative relationships with more experienced researchers to hone their skills and maximize the potential for meaningful research findings (Schaefer et al., 2011). This said, all educational institutions are encouraged to engage in research that improves and supports their curricula. Educational research cannot and should not be seen as a role for only large research institutions. Students attending institutions that primarily focus on teaching also deserve educational experiences with known efficacy.

ADVANTAGES OF CONDUCTING RESEARCH IN VIRTUAL AND GAME-BASED ENVIRONMENTS

There are a number of advantages to conducting research using simulation in general. Researchers can follow and evaluate subjects and learners' actions as they work their way though complex clinical situations without any risk occurring to patients because the patient is represented as a physical mannikin or as either a PC or NPC existing as digital phenomenon. Research using simulation has the potential to glean important information about human behavior in complex clinical environments. It also allows educators to make assessments about student cognitive and behavioral gain and change that are not possible in actual clinical environments due to ethical considerations and situational availability.

Nursing students, medical and other clinical sciences students may complete their entire undergraduate training without ever seeing a cardiac resuscitation. Simulations broaching this topic not only provide an important learning opportunity for students, but also provide educators and administrators with important information about how novices will react when responding to clinical crisis situations. This sort of research proposition simply is not possible in actual clinical environments where the most qualified clinician must take charge as a matter of ethical imperative to effectuate the best possible outcome during clinical crises (Bauman, 2007; Hammond, 2004).

Simulations taking place in fixed laboratories and even in situ often take advantage of sophisticated computer modeling software and video capture that allows researchers to collect data in ways often not possible in real-world clinical settings. Software data collection matrixes allow for the automatic data collection of things such as modeled physiology and even some tactile events, such as pulse checks when completed by subjects. Researchers can video record behavioral aspects of subjects for further analysis.

Research occurring in digital spaces may not be able to attend to tactile or haptic elements of actual clinical spaces, but can provide matrixes that allow for much more consistent data collection than actual clinical spaces and even fixed-space simulation laboratories. Researchers can engineer matrixes for data collection into digital spaces as a matter of environmental design. Data collection matrixes can include data such as time on task, time off task, time in environment, and number of attempts to completion of task. In automated digital environments this data is precise because a researcher has engineered the element of human error out of the data collection process.

Digital spaces designed for educational purposes can move beyond student evaluation in the traditional didactic sense. Behavioral and cognitive aspects of game play may lead to the development of research questions and hypotheses and even elements of curriculum and instructional design. As discussed in detail in the previous chapter, we can leverage commercial video games and virtual environments originally produced for entertainment purposes for educational purposes. We argue that we can use existing commercial spaces for clinical education and for educational research in the clinical sciences.

Confounding Variables, Time, and Location

We can mitigate challenges related to time, location, and confounding variables when collecting data in digital environments, particularly when using persistent environments that we access through the Internet. One of the challenges associated with research validity is that it can be very difficult to realistically generalize study results beyond the discrete population being studied. Further, internal validity is affected by the consistency of how we implement research protocol throughout the study.

Additional Confounding Variables

Confounding variables can threaten internal and external validity even when conducting simulation-based investigations occurring in relatively controlled fixed laboratories. Controlling confounding variables is one of the major challenges associated with educational, particularly experiential, research (Ewert & Sibthorp, 2009) (Table 9.1).

Interruption of research protocols during data collection is a very real problem when collecting data in actual practice environments. It can be so confounding that such interruptions may corrupt data collected in actual practice environments. We may be unable to use corrupted data or data collected under unusual circumstances that does not adhere research protocols. When data are collected using in situ simulation in an actual clinical space, like an emergency department, the dynamics of the rest of the unit are likely going to affect and even interrupt data collection. When similar research protocols are implemented in a fixed-space, mannikin-based laboratory, investigators are better able to control for interruptions and the confounding variables of a dynamic workspace. However, the fixed-space laboratory, even when providing a high level of environmental fidelity has its limitations in terms of reach of the physical space. For example, in some cases if a subject leaves the room, they entirely remove themselves from the simulation.

In digital environments we can minimize and possibly eliminate interruptions. We can design environmental fidelity to exist beyond the confines of any one screenshot or room. Furthermore, we can control variables introduced to the simulation scenario so that each simulation or clinical scenario for each subject in the cohort being evaluated is consistent. Consistency is a key element to promoting internal validity.

Time

Time is a valuable commodity for educators, researchers, and students. Educators, particularly those teaching in clinical roles are often pressed to find enough time to adequately prepare for their students and make vital decisions about student clinical readiness and safety. It is not uncommon for clinical faculty across the clinical disciplines to arrive at clinical sites hours in advance of students and remain long after students have left.

TABLE 9.1

Threat Assessment Related to Research of Internal and External Validity Among Fixed, In Situ, and Digital Environments

Example of Confounding Variable	Fixed Laboratory	In Situ	Digital Environment	External Validity	Internal Validity
Interruption to research protocol	Easily controlled and unlikely to occur	Likely to occur and likely to occur	Easily controlled and unlikely to occur	Minimal threat	Significant threat
Researcher bias or variation among those implementing the protocol	Likely to occur if multiple people are implementing the research protocol	Likely to occur if multiple people are implementing the research protocol	Unlikely to occur, particularly if the research protocol has been automated	Minimal-to-moderate threat	Significant threat
Homogeneous sample	Likely to occur	Likely to occur	Subject recruitment outside of a given geographical area is easily facilitated	Moderate-to-severe threat	Minimal threat
Time/availability of research staff or subjects	Likely to occur	Likely to occur	Unlikely to occur, particularly if the research protocol has been automated	Moderate-to-severe threat	Moderate-to-severe threat
Inconsistency of data collection	Somewhat likely to occur	Likely to occur	Unlikely to occur, particularly if the research protocol has been automated	Moderate-to-severe threat	Moderate-to-severe threat

217

Those engaging in research often have multiple duties at their institutions. It is rare for those working in clinical or teaching capacities to have protected time set aside and specifically reserved for research. Yet at many institutions, engaging in research is seen as an expected step toward professional development. Crafting, executing, and reporting the results of research projects is hard and time-consuming work. Contributing to a body of scientific literature in a meaningful way so that findings are available to others in a translational way can be difficult.

Research around mannikin-based simulation is challenging because time is a tangible variable that researchers must account for. Unless the research you are conducting exists within a curriculum, scheduling additional time for students and support staff to be in the lab can be a daunting task with monetary consequences. Many simulation laboratories have cost per hour and cost per student built into their operational plans. Further, asking students to volunteer as subjects in research represents a time commitment that cannot be ethically coerced. If students or subjects perceive participation as inconvenient, threatening, or not worth their time, they can and will opt out of participation.

Location

Location and time are related variables in terms of accomplishing research goals. Collecting data for research projects often involves the investigator going to the subjects or the subjects coming to the investigator. In the case of mannikin-based simulation research, the most likely scenario is that research subjects come to the simulation laboratory to participate in the research protocol. Even though mannikin-based simulators are often portable, they are expensive and can be difficult to transport to remote facilities. For example, even modest high-fidelity mannikin simulators cost $30,000 to $100,000. It may not be acceptable to the research institution to transport simulators in private vehicles. Researchers have to make simulators with appropriate support staff available that support research protocols where and when subjects are available.

In a recent countywide advanced airway placement study using a task trainer and an endoscope to evaluate laryngeal mask airway (LMA) placement among paramedics, the following resources and logistics were required to secure a convenience sample of 35 participants among some 160 possible subjects. Investigators comprised of a research registered nurse and anesthesiologist made four trips into the community with the airway task trainer, endoscope, LMAs, and other supplies needed to facilitate the research protocol. Aside from the cost of the research supplies, the research teams were removed from clinical and teaching responsibilities to collect the data for this investigation. The conservative cost of completing this very small research project was between $5,000 and $10,000 (Bauman, Joffe, Liew, & Seider,

2009). While this study would not lend itself to a virtual environment it does illustrate how even small research projects have a cost associated with them, which is time and location dependent.

Seeking research opportunities in virtual and game-based environments have the advantage of control. While it is difficult to account for all confounding variables, virtual environments can be designed to exert control in ways not possible in real world or created spaces such as simulation laboratories. The virtual world redefines the time and location paradigm. Continuous online or digital spaces are persistent and exist and can be made accessible without regard to conventional working hours. These environments are available wherever subjects can access the Internet. Further, because virtual environments are designed to be intuitive and can include programmed mechanisms for data collection and are less fragile than mannikin-based simulators, they may require no co-presence of research staff at the point of data collection.

Consider a clinical risk or threat assessment game that exists in a persistent online virtual environment. The objective of the game is to identify environmental risks that affect patient safety. The problem statement associated with the related research project discusses the implication of patient falls in an inpatient clinical environment. The research question might ask, does providing game-based training on risk management related to patient falls affect the number of patient falls over time?. The hypothesis for this research project says playing and completing the game will decrease the incidence of falls. For this sort of game, the independent variable can be accessed at the convenience of the subjects anywhere they have Internet access without regard for time. Additional useful information related to time in environment and time on task are collected remotely and automatically.

While this is a simple example, it emphasizes how we can use a game-based intervention to facilitate translational research that is both educational and clinical in nature. From the educational perspective, subjects learn about risks and hazards that cause patient falls. From a patient safety perspective, the intervention has the potential to increase clinician awareness and get them to decrease fall risks and hazards thereby decreasing patient falls.

RESEARCH ON HUMAN SUBJECTS

IRB regulations are becoming more strict regarding evaluation research as well as clinical research involving patients (Oakes, 2002) and human subjects in general. Also, more and more journals require that authors state the status of ethics approval of their research as requirement for publishing (Amdur & Biddle, 1997). It is thus incumbent upon researchers conducting research on teaching methods and tools to conform to local, national, and international ethical guidelines for conducting research and to be particularly aware of issues that may be unique to conducting research using virtual and game-based teaching tools.

Committees that review and approve research in the United States are typically referred to as Institutional Review Boards (IRBs), Independent Ethics Committees (IECs), or Ethical Review Boards (ERBs). There are also independent IRBs in the United States that are not connected to institutions. These are often used by commercial firms such as marketing companies and companies that provide goods and services to the healthcare industry that seek to do research with human subjects. In Europe, the equivalent of the IRB is the Ethics Committee. International, national, local, and institutional guidelines bear on the actions and decisions of individual IRBs.

Ethical Principles that Guide IRBs

In general, IRBs evaluate research based on ethical principles of respect, beneficence, and justice (National Commission for the Protection of Human Subjects of Biomedical and Behavioral Research, 1978). They support the principle of respect by ensuring that participants in research studies understand their rights as individuals to decline participation or freely volunteer to participate. In particular, they seek to protect populations whose autonomy may be compromised (children, incarcerated individuals, and patients) and therefore may feel coerced to participate in research studies. Students in classes that are a part of research on education can be considered vulnerable populations if their participation in research appears to be a mandatory part of class (Roberts, Geppert, Connor, Nguyen, & Warner, 2001).

IRBs also review research based on the principle of beneficence by making sure that no harm is done to participants and that researchers maximize the benefits associated with conducting the research (such as determining an effective training tool) in relation to possible risks of study participation (such as in-class knowledge gains compromised to serve the goals of the research study). IRBs will review studies to make sure these risks are balanced and managed so that potential harm will be addressed appropriately. IRBs will also be particularly sensitive to research conducted that captures personal information in a digital form (as opposed to only on paper) and can place participant confidentially at risk because it can easily be transferred and distributed broadly. Many digital learning technologies have the capacity to capture and store vast amounts of data that can be stored digitally. Because confidentiality can be so easily compromised, researchers should be prepared ahead of time to take measures to minimize these risks with digital teaching technologies.

Guided by the principle of justice, IRBs also review research to make sure that it benefits advantaged as well as disadvantaged subgroups in a population. This can mean that the research proposed should demonstrate that the sample recruited for a study will be representative of the people who will benefit and if certain subgroups will not be represented, that there are compelling reasons for this situation. All of these ethical principles are outlined in more detail in the Belmont Report (National Commission for the Protection of Human Subjects of Biomedical and Behavioral Research, 1978).

Given the diversity of guidelines and settings of IRBs, familiarity with your appropriate IRB for your research study should be planned for well in advance of the desired date one would like to begin collecting data. Institutions can vary greatly in the time it will take to approve studies (Stair, Reed, Radeos, Koski, & Camargo, 2001), even studies that pose minimal risks to participants (Hirshon et al., 2002). Review and approval time may also be dependent on how often IRBs meet, the average number of issues to be addressed in the application, and the researcher's ability to address the concerns identified by the IRB in a satisfactory time and manner. Good planning and preparation in regard to IRB approval is well worth the effort. The timing and requirements of one's local IRB should be sought well in advance so that IRB approval is obtained in a timely manner and does not negatively effect opportunities for data collection.

Even if a research project seems to qualify for exemption from ethics review because an educator or researcher believes the research protocol presents virtually no risk to human participants, the IRB ultimately decides whether or not the research is exempt from review. There is some suggestion in the literature that many educators wrongly assume that their research on curriculum effectiveness with pre- and posttesting on students enrolled in their curriculum is exempt from ethics review (Tomkowiak & Gunderson, 2004). If questions arise, most IRBs are very open to direct contact with applicants BEFORE the application is due because they are also interested in minimizing misunderstandings and addressing problems before they reach the review board. Further, even if a research project qualifies for exemption under one of several categories, the exemption status is ultimately the decision of the IRB. Substantial and career-damaging implications may be warranted and imposed on researchers who do not comply with IRB processes.

Here are some practical steps to take in seeking ethics approval for a research study:

1. *Find out where you need to apply.* Some institutions have healthcare and non-healthcare ethics reviews committees. Research on educational tools and processes is something that does not involve patients so that a non-healthcare review may be appropriate. On the other hand, if the study is conducted in a hospital, nursing school, medical school, or across clinical disciplines the institution may require that the study receive approval from the health sciences or related ethics board. If the research is being conducted by a for-profit training company, the company may use the services of a commercial review board that is independent of educational institutions

to review their research. It is very possible, even likely that research proposals may need approval from multiple IRBs, particularly if the research will require collaboration among researchers from multiple institutions or subjects will be evaluated at multiple institutions.

2. *Find out when you will need to apply.* IRBs usually have a website where they post submission deadlines for applications and meeting dates when they review received applications. Often different types of applications are reviewed on varying schedules. For example, minimal risk and exemption applications may be reviewed on a continual basis, while more complex applications might be reviewed monthly or quarterly. What is not often published is when they will get their comments to you, how long you have to address their comments and make changes, and when they will meet next to review your changes. Make sure you know this so you can avoid disappointments and potentially costly delays in data collection. Keep in mind that it may be difficult for IRBs to evaluate research on new technologies that they do not understand and this may cause delays in the process. For example, when submitting an application that explicitly uses the term "patient" when describing an avatar-based encounter in a virtual or digital environment, you must make sure that the reviewers understand that no real patient will be put at risk and that any actual patient data used to create the virtual patient being represented as a digital phenomenon has been stripped of any identifying information. Further, you must assure the IRB that all local and federal guidelines such as the Health Insurance Portability and Accountability Act rules have been followed as it relates to using actual patient records and information when creating virtual patients and related simulations. In a related example, when submitting a research proposal related to evaluating students interacting within a mannikin-based simulation laboratory, very specific language related to the description of the simulator was requested by the IRB. Clarification was required to assure the IRB that the patient, represented by a high-fidelity mannikin was free of any human or animal biological tissue (Bauman, 2007).

3. *Write your application.* Because the timing of IRB approval processes forces many researchers to apply for ethics approval early, they often have to submit research protocols that are not fully finalized. This is not ideal but virtually every IRB has a process for submitting and gaining approval for amendments and changes to your research protocol. This also has to be submitted and approved on time. In general though, it is easier to submit an amendment rather than a complete protocol so it pays to go ahead and submit for approval early. Researchers should be aware that IRBs will require amendments to add or remove key personnel from applications. If there are changes in your research team it is imperative that the proper amendment is provided to the IRB and that you can demonstrate that those being added to the research team are qualified to engage in research involving human subjects. Requirements and qualifications for participating

as a researcher will be established by individual IRBs. Nonqualified individuals are generally prohibited from active participation on the research team.

4. *Contact the IRB with any questions you might have.* If you are not sure how to fill out a form or how much information to put in your consent form, do not hesitate to call the IRB. They will not be able to tell you exactly what to say, but they can provide helpful guidance. The IRB will help you determine what type of category you should be filing for. A full IRB review is very comprehensive and time consuming to prepare. Further, some IRBs require a substantial filing fee for full reviews. However, an exemption application may be relatively easy to submit and may not have an associated filing fee. This said, posing thoughtful questions to the IRB would help you make these types of determinations.

5. *Submit your protocol on time.* Make sure you have all the documents they ask for, the required signatures, and funds ready for payment if your IRB requires this for a review. Keep in mind that submitting an on-time and complete application will likely require the collaboration of multiple people in your organization or department. When grant money is involved or fees must be paid you may need signatures and promissory letters from department chairs, deans, and various other administrators.

6. *Address comments and requests for changes from the IRB.* If you did not receive a letter with comments and requests for changes, skip to the next step. It is very likely, however, that you will receive a number of comments and requests for changes from the IRB. Make sure you address them by the deadline and deal with them in a professional way. If some of the comments seem irrational or picky, keep in mind that people from different backgrounds sit on review boards. No matter what, they are all trying to do their job as best they can and they are often not paid for the work they do. They deserve to be treated with the same high level of respect that you will show your research subjects. Again, if you have trouble answering the questions, call the IRB for guidance or consult with people who are more experienced with the IRB review process. Reiterate this process until you gain approval. Many larger departments and institutions have dedicated staff to help researchers prepare research proposals and navigate the IRB process. You should seek out these people and ask for their advice. Experienced researchers and staff specifically trained in human subjects research will be able to help you expedite the IRB approval process.

7. *File the approval letter and get ready to do your study!* If your submission was approved with no comments or requests for changes, you should file your letter away and get ready for the actual work of conducting your study. You should also celebrate this situation because it happens very rarely. To this point, you should not be discouraged when clarifications or further explanation is requested from the IRB. Receiving requests for more information or modification of your research proposal is common.

8. *File any revisions or changes to your protocol to the IRB.* Major changes to your protocol and especially your consent form need to be approved before you enact those changes in your study. The IRB should be consulted to confirm what kinds of changes they require to undergo review before actually submitting the revisions.

9. *Make reports as required by your IRB.* Depending on how long a research study takes to carry out, IRBs usually ask for regular reports of the progress of the study and also for a final report once the study is completed. They are typically fairly simple to fill out and complete and allow the IRB to monitor the progress of studies. Failing to comply with required reports can lead to a suspension of your research protocol and sanctions placed on the primary investigator and the rest of the research team.

The IRB process is a requirement for studies involving human subjects. This section outlined the principles that guide the work of the IRBs, issues that researchers proposing studies using virtual and game approaches to clinical education should keep in mind, and general steps that are involved in working with IRB in conducting research with human subjects.

Case Study: Examining the Complexity of In-World Data Analysis

A methodological challenge of conducting data evaluation from studies that involve multiple participants interacting in a virtual world like *Second Life* is the painstaking process needed to analyze each participant's interaction and contribution. In environments like *Second Life* every avatar has total control of their in-world location, camera view angles, zoom level, and objects to interact with. When using just the researcher's point of view it is only possible to capture some portions of the interaction process occurring within the digital environment. Inevitably some important interactions occurring in the environment are likely to be missed.

The challenge associated with capturing important interactions with objects and other avatars in digital immersive worlds consists of programmatically embedding code into each interactive object that players/subjects will or are likely to interact with. This programmatic approach automatically keeps track of the number of times that in-world objects are manipulated; by whom and the exact time the interaction took place. For instance, Montoya, Massey, and Lockwood (2011) explored the link between collaborative behaviors and team performance in a 3-D cube puzzle-solving task in *Second Life* using script logs to record the contribution of each participant during the research protocol. The interactions recorded through the script included, among others, the number of times each participant "touched" a 3-D cube, which initiated the process to start solving a new puzzle as well as the number of times each participant clicked on a button that indicated that the team believed that a puzzle was solved.

While we can use log scripting to document and evaluate the process of user-interface interaction within virtual worlds, it has several drawbacks. The amount of time and knowledge required to write and test each script can be very time consuming. Further, log scripting may be limited in the type of environment interaction that it can accurately record. In general, this type of data capture document's the result of an interaction but not the reason why that interaction took or did not take place. Studies in which it is paramount to analyze each participant's experience and their motives for interaction within a virtual or game-based space require the video capture of each participant's screen to accurately detail each participant's in-world interaction. Techniques like stimulated recall could then be used by having each participant narrate one's own experience while watching their own recorded experience (Appelman, 2007).

The use of specialized applications to record the screen and participants' verbal communication while immersed in a digital environment requires computing resources capable of simultaneously capturing complex applications including: screencast software itself to record the screen and the virtual world program in which the participants' interaction takes place. Software must be configured so that in-world communication can take place in real time and so that audiovisual capture of in-world interactions is of value to the researchers. In a sense, using this type of capture is akin to making animated movies. While this seems to be a very basic function, even those working in fixed mannikin-based simulation laboratories can attest to the challenges of capturing usable audio and visual components during simulations.

An investigation facing some of the challenges described above is a dissertation study currently being conducted in the School of Education of a large Midwestern university. One of the goals of the study is to explore the patterns of collaboration that take place when two participants, physically apart from each other, play an instructional game called the "Diffusion Simulation Game" (DSG) (Lara, Myers, Frick, Aslan, & Michaelidou, 2010). This game teaches concepts and strategies related to Rogers' (2003) Diffusion of Innovations theory. The original online version of this game was adapted for play in *Second Life* using the co-browsing capabilities that this virtual world provides.

In the DSG collaborative version, two players need to join efforts to persuade teachers from a fictitious high school to adopt an instructional innovation by conducting specific diffusion activities (Figure 9.2). Both players can see each other's interaction with the game; however, unlike common screen sharing through a videoconferencing application, the DSG interface allows for one player to individually inspect elements of the game while the other player inspects different elements. For instance, a player could analyze the social networks of the teachers in the school while the other player is examining the role of teachers' committee assignments.

To analyze the individual contribution and participation in the collaboration process in the DSG study, screencast software is used to record each

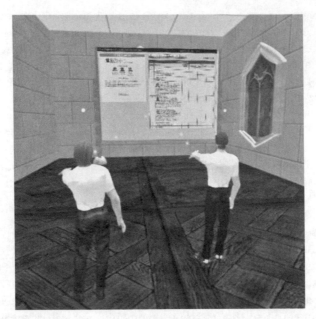

FIGURE 9.2
Playing the diffusion simulation game collaboratively

participant's screen and voice. The screen recordings from both participants are then played side by side to observe what exactly each participant was seeing, doing, and saying during their game play. By incrementing the number of participants taking part in the study, the technology requirements and the complexity of data analysis also increases.

The point of this case study is not to discourage novice researchers; rather it is to get them to be forward thinking about how they will engage the research process as it relates to games and simulation. As technology advances, methods and techniques for data capture within digital environments will improve. Recall the virtual environment provides the opportunity for types of research that simply are not possible in actual clinical environments, but may map translational effect in the real world.

SUMMARY

In this chapter we emphasized the importance of educational research arguing that all schools, programs, and institutions have an obligation to evaluate new teaching tools and technology including games and simulations before, during, and after integration into new and existing curricula. From this perspective, research should be seen as a continuous quality improvement process. Some will move beyond the educational continuous quality improvement role and develop robust programs of research focused on simulation and game-based learning using multimedia environments like virtual world learning spaces. The entire spectrum of research adds to the scientific literature and builds expertise in the still relatively new genre of multimedia and game-based educational research particularly within the scope of clinical education.

We discussed the advantages of conducting research in immersive virtual worlds. We paid specific attention to time and place. We believe that the virtual world represents a powerful paradigm shift in how education will be delivered and how research that supports nursing and other types of clinical education will occur. We also discussed the potential advantages of using the digital learning spaces for educational research from the perspective of control and mitigation of confounding variable, arguing that virtual spaces may offer a degree of control not available in actual clinical environments or fixed space simulation centers.

We also provided a very brief review of research methodology and key research terms. Specifically, we briefly discussed quantitative and qualitative research methodology and several key elements of these research processes. We discussed the importance of following a thoughtful research plan and emphasized the importance of internal and external validity. The IRB process, an integral part of behavioral research and any type of research involving human subjects was detailed. When possible, explicit examples were provided to illustrate and emphasize our discussion and importance of the IRB process.

Finally, we provided a brief case study to illustrate some of the challenges associated with conducting research in digital environments, specifically repurposed digital environments like *Second Life*. This case study is meant to be thought provoking, not discouraging. Throughout the chapter we urged novice researchers to seek mentors who can guide and support them through the research process. Further, we urge more experienced investigators to provide mentorship to novice researchers.

Research worth doing almost always comes with challenges. Conducting research is in itself formative. Understanding the process and the resources needed to develop and advance a research project or more comprehensive program should be exciting and motivating. We believe that as researchers explore the digital world from a scientific perspective they will contribute to the literature and drive best practices in ways that inform educational practice and in turn clinical practice and patient outcome. In order to establish external validity for simulation and game-based learning that provides a documented translational effect, we urge the curious to take on the role of researcher. We emphasize that this role is just as important for those working in small organizations, programs, and schools as it is for those working in larger research institutions. Research drives and justifies curriculum. As we begin to integrate simulation and game-based learning into nursing and health sciences curricula, it is imperative that we make curriculum content and delivery decisions based on sound analysis of data.

REFERENCES

Akl, E. A., Pretorius, R. W., Sackett, K., Erdley, W. S., Bhoopathi, P. S., Alfarah, Z. et al. (2010). The effect of educational games on medical students' learning outcomes: A systematic review: BEME Guide No 14. *Medical Teacher, 32*(1), 16–27. doi:10.3109/01421590903473969

Amdur, R. J., & Biddle, C. (1997). Institutional Review Board approval and publication of human research results. *JAMA: The Journal of the American Medical Association, 277*(11), 909–914. doi: 10.1001/jama.1997.03540350059034

Appelman, R. (2007). Experiential modes of game play. Situated Play, Proceedings of DiGRA 2007 Conference. Retrieved January 25, 2012, from http://www.digra.org/dl/db/07311.16497.pdf

Bandura, A. (2004). Health promotion by social cognitive means. *Health Education and Behavior, 31*(2), 143–164. doi: 10.1177/1090198104263660

Bauman, E. (2007). *High fidelity simulation in healthcare.* PhD dissertation, The University of Wisconsin-Madison, United States. Dissertations & Theses @ CIC Institutions database (Publication no. AAT 3294196 ISBN: 9780549383109 ProQuest document ID: 1453230861).

Bauman, E. B., Joffe, A. M., Liew, E. C., & Seider, S. P. (2009). Simulation-based training to teach paramedics how to place and intubate through the single use LMA-Fastrach™ [peer reviewed scientific poster abstract]. *Simulation in Healthcare, 4*(4), 244.

Ben-Zur, H., Yagil, D., & Spitzer, A. (1999). Evaluation of an innovative curriculum: Nursing education in the next century. *Journal of Advanced Nursing, 30*(6), 1432–1440.

Brown, S. J., Lieberman, D. A., Gemeny, B. A., Fan, Y. C., Wilson, D. M., & Pasta, D. J. (1997). Educational video game for juvenile diabetes: Results of a controlled trial. *Informatics for Health and Social Care, 22*(1), 77–89. doi: doi:10.3109/14639239709089835

Campbell, D. T., & Stanley, J. C. (1963). *Experimental and quasi-experimental designs for research.* Chicago: Rand McNally.

Cane, V. R., & Heim, A. W. (1950). The effects of repeated retesting: III. Further experiments and general conclusions. *Quarterly Journal of Experimental Psychology, 2*(4), 182–197. doi: 10.1080/17470215008416596

Commission on Collegiate Nursing Education. (2009). *Standards for Accreditation: Baccalaureate and graduate and degree nursing programs.* Commission on Collegiate Nursing Education. Washington DC.

Cook, T. D., & Campbell, D. T. (1979). *Quasi-experimentation: Design and analysis for field settings.* Boston: Houghton Mifflin.

Diekelmann, N. L. (Ed.). (2003). *Teaching the practitioners of care: New pedagogies for the health professions.* Madison, WI: The University of Wisconsin Press.

Ewert, A., & Sibthorp, J. (2009). Creating outcomes through experiential education: The challenge of confounding variable. *Journal of Experiential Education, 31*(3), 376–389.

Guy, S., Ratzki-Leewing, A., & Gwadry-Sridhar, F. (2011). Moving beyond the stigma: Systematic review of video games and their potential to combat obesity. *International Journal of Hypertension, 2011*, 1–13. doi: 10.4061/2011/179124.

Hammond, J. (2004). Simulation in critical care and trauma education and training. *Current Opinion Critical Care, 10*(5), 325–329.

Hirshon, J. M., Krugman, S. D., Witting, M. D., Furuno, J. P., Limcangco, M. R., Perisse, A. R. et al. (2002). Variability in Institutional Review Board Assessment of minimal-risk research. *Academic Emergency Medicine, 9*(12), 1417–1420. doi: 10.1197/aemj.9.12.1417

Kato, P. M. (2010). Video games in health care: Closing the gap. *Review of General Psychology, 14*(2), 113–121.

Kato, P. M. (2012a). Evaluating efficacy and validating games for health. *Games for Health Journal, 1*(1). doi: 10.1089/g4h.2012.1017.

Kato, P. M. (2012b). The role of the researcher in making effective serious games for health. In S. Arnab, I. Dunwell, & K. Debattista (Eds.), *Serious games for health-care: Applications and implications*. Hershey, PA: IGI Global.

Kato, P. M., Cole, S. W., Bradlyn, A. S., & Pollock, B. H. (2008). A video game improves behavioral outcomes in adolescents and young adults with cancer: A randomized trial. *Pediatrics, 122*(2), e305–e317. doi: 10.1542/peds.2007-3134

Kulik, J. A., Kulik, C.-L. C., & Bangert, R. L. (1984). Effects of practice on aptitude and achievement test scores. *American Educational Research Journal, 21*(2), 435–447. doi: 10.3102/00028312021002435

Lara, M., Myers, R. D., Frick, T. W., Aslan, S., & Michaelidou, T. (2010). A design case: Developing an enhanced version of the diffusion simulation game. *International Journal of Designs for Learning, 1*(1). Retrieved January 25, 2012, from http://scholarworks.iu.edu/journals/index.php/ijdl/index

Marascuilo, R. A., & Serlin, R. C. (1988). *Statistical methods for the social and behavioral sciences*. New York: W. H. Freeman.

Mawn, B., & Reece, S. M. (2000). Reconfiguring the curriculum for the new millennium: The process of change. *Journal of Nursing Education, 39*(3), 101–108.

Montoya, M. M., Massey, A. P., & Lockwood, N. S. (2011). 3D Collaborative virtual environments: Exploring the link between collaborative behaviors and team performance. *Decision Sciences, 42*(2), 451–476.

National Commission for the Protection of Human Subjects of Biomedical and Behavioral Research. (1978). *The Belmont Report: Ethical principles and guidelines for the protection of human subjects of research*. Washington, DC: U.S. Government Printing Office.

Nishisaki, A., Keren, R., & Nadkarni, V. (2007). Does simulation improve patient safety?: Self-efficacy, competence, operational performance, and patient safety. *Anesthesiology Clinics, 25*(2), 225–236. doi: 10.1016/j.anclin.2007.03.009

Oakes, J. M. (2002). Risks and wrongs in social science research. *Evaluation Review, 26*(5), 443–479. doi: 10.1177/019384102236520

Polit, D. F., & Hungler, B. P. (1999). *Nursing research: Principles and methods* (6th ed.). Philadelphia: Lippincott.

Randel, J. M., Morris, B. A., Wetzel, C. D., & Whitehill, B. V. (1992). The effectiveness of games for educational purposes: A review of recent research. *Simulation & Gaming, 23*(3), 261–276. doi: 10.1177/1046878192233001

Roberts, L. W., Geppert, C., Connor, R., Nguyen, K., & Warner, T. D. (2001). An invitation for medical educators to focus on ethical and policy issues in research and scholarly practice. *Academic Medicine, 76*(9), 876–885.

Rogers, E. M. (2003). *Elements of diffusion*. In E. M. Rogers (Ed.), *Diffusion of innovations* (5th ed.). New York: The Free Press.

Rothwell, P. M. (2005). External validity of randomised controlled trials?: To whom do the results of this trial apply? *The Lancet*, *365*(9453), 82–93.

Salthouse, T. A., Schroeder, D. H., & Ferrer, E. (2004). Estimating retest effects in longitudinal assessments of cognitive functioning in adults between 18 and 60 years of age. *Developmental Psychology*, *40*(5), 813–822.

Schaefer, J., III, Vanderbilt, A., Cason, C., Bauman, E., Glavin, R., Lee, F. et al. (2011). Literature review: Instructional design and pedagogy science in healthcare simulation. *Simulation in Healthcare*, *6*(7), S30–S41.

Stair, T. O., Reed, C. R., Radeos, M. S., Koski, G., & Camargo, C. A. (2001). Variation in Institutional Review Board responses to a standard protocol for a multicenter clinical trial. *Academic Emergency Medicine*, *8*(6), 636–641. doi: 10.1111/j.1553-2712.2001.tb00177.x

Tomkowiak, J. M., & Gunderson, A. J. (2004). To IRB or not to IRB? *Academic Medicine*, *79*(7), 628–632.

Appendix of Resources/Products

ALLAN BARCLAY, BETHANY BRYANT, AND GERALD STAPLETON

HEALTHCARE EDUCATION IN *SECOND LIFE*

Ann Meyers Medical Center

*T*he AMMC is currently focused on information and education regarding health, especially women's health issues. The project has interactive exhibits related to research, treatment, and prevention of cervical cancer and other conditions as well as facilities for nursing and medical education.

Web: http://ammc.wordpress.com/
Second Life: http://maps.secondlife.com/secondlife/Fashion Boulevard II/164/96/43

Biomedicine Research Labs: SBARRO Health Research Organization

SHRO is an international organization that focuses on finding cures for cancer, cardiovascular and other diseases by identifying their underlying molecular mechanisms. In the real world, SHRO has facilities in Philadelphia, Pennsylvania and in Siena, Italy. Their virtual world headquarters in *Second Life* provides an opportunity to share their research findings with an international audience in an interactive format which includes exhibits and meeting facilities.

Web: www.shro.org
Second Life: http://maps.secondlife.com/secondlife/Biomedicine Research Labs/70/97/22

Evergreen Hospital: Tacoma Community College

By using *Second Life* avatars, John Miller, RN and the faculty at Tacoma Community College can present students in the health professions with virtual patients of any age, ethnicity, personal characteristics, and medical condition. The virtual patient's actions, communication, and vital signs can be controlled to create a simulated patient encounter either standardized or customized for each student. Students practice their skill in case management and patient communication by interacting with both the virtual patient and medical devices as well as communicating among the members of the healthcare team.

Web: http://jsmillerrn.blogspot.com/
Video: www.youtube.com/watch?v=oLhuBNkYOsU
Second Life: http://maps.secondlife.com/secondlife/Evergreen Island 3/34/ 170/30

Imperial College of London

This project has been developed by the Faculty of Medicine and was originally funded by a grant from the Joint Integration Systems Committee (JISC) in the EU. Game-based learning activities are provided to allow medical students working individually or in groups to examine and diagnose virtual patients. The students must select from a bank of tests to help them determine the correct diagnosis. The project involves an integration of the virtual world of *Second Life* with the Moodle course management system.

Web: www.imperial.ac.uk
Second Life: http://maps.secondlife.com/secondlife/Imperial College London/ 148/65/27

NewWorld Initiative for Clinician Education

This project has been developed by Gerald Stapleton at the University of Illinois at Chicago College of Medicine for the purpose of investigating the use of virtual environments to facilitate learning in the health care professions. Focusing on communications skills, the initiative has developed scenarios in which physician trainees interact with actors who are trained to serve as standardized patients and with virtual patients programmed and controlled by an external computer using artificial intelligence (AIML). Similar projects have also been developed with the same name on the open simulator-based virtual worlds New World Grid (www.newworldgrid.com) and The Health Grid (www.thehealthgrid.org).

Web: www.newworldclinic.com
Video (Student Recruitment): http://go.uic.edu/avatar
Second Life: http://maps.secondlife.com/secondlife/Erudio Consortio/190/ 70/25

Nightingale Isle

A place where healthcare professionals can hang out, have fun, and learn. Jone Tiffany DNP, Associate Professor of Nursing at Bethel College, maintains this project. This project is dedicated to distance learning through the use of virtual worlds and will eventually support an ambulatory clinic, birthing center, and education area.

Web: www.nightingaleisleblogspot.com
Second Life: http://maps.secondlife.com/secondlife/Nightingale%20Isle/109/128/21

Ohio State Medical Center

Doug Danforth, PhD and his colleagues in the Department of Obstetrics and Gynecology at Ohio State have created interactive models of the human testis and ovary that allow students to "tour" these organs to develop a more thorough understanding of their design and function.

Web: www.biolreprod.org/cgi/content/meeting_abstract/78/1_Meeting Abstracts/129-b
Video: www.youtube.com/watch?v=vEk48Sc9UaM
Second Life: http://maps.secondlife.com/secondlife/OSU   Medicine/211/132/26

Postpartum Hemorrhage Management: Boise State University and University of Auckland

This project was created by Scott Diener, PhD of the University of Auckland, New Zealand. Students attend to actors known as standardized patients who are trained to portray patients with various medical conditions. The SPs, in turn, evaluate the students and provide feedback to help the students improve their clinical skills. In a collaboration between Aukland and Boise State University in Idaho, nursing students work in groups to practice their skills in dealing with issues involved with incidents of obstetric hemorrhage.

Video: www.healthinformaticsforum.com/video/university-of-auckland-in (Overview)
Video: www.youtube.com/watch?v=G2jN7L80bH8&feature=related (Nursing Scenario)
Second Life: http://maps.secondlife.com/secondlife/Long White Cloud/108/71/27

SL Healthy

SL Healthy is a web-based resource center created by Patricia Anderson, Emerging Technologies Librarian from the University of Michigan providing information and links to health and health education resources in *Second Life*.

Web: http://slhealthy.wetpaint.com

Tox Town (National Library of Medicine)

Tox Town has been developed by the National Library of Medicine to provide information on toxic chemicals in the environment and how these chemicals impact human health. The information found on the site is based on the TOXNET and MedlinePlus resources from the NLM. A heads-up display (HUD) is available to assist in the use of interactive functionality built into the project.

Web: http://towtown.nlm.nih.gov
Second Life: http://maps.secondlife.com/secondlife/Virtual NLM/113/134/25

UW Oshkosh College of Nursing

Students in the Accelerated BSN Program interact with scripted patient avatars in scenarios which simulate high-risk but low-volume clinical experiences such as myocardial infarctions, hemorrhages, or cerebral vascular accidents allowing the students to practice procedures, receive formative feedback, and make corrections while avoiding risk to real-life patients.

Web: www.uwosh.edu/con/undergraduate-bsn/accelerated-online-bachelors-to-bsn
Video: www.youtube.com/watch?v=oReztkUkpGI&feature=related
Second Life: http://maps.secondlife.com/secondlife/OshCON/131/57/44

Virtual Ability Island

This project provides information and support for individuals with real-life disabilities and other newcomers to *Second Life*. It is recognized for its award-winning accessible orientation course based on the Universal Design standards.

Web: www.virtualability.org/
Second Life: http://slurl.com/secondlife/Virtual Ability/129/128/23

HEALTHCARE GAMES AND SIMULATIONS

3-D Brain www.dnalc.org/	Use the touch screen on your iPhone or iPod to rotate and zoom around 29 interactive structures. Discover how each brain region functions, what happens when it is injured, and how it is involved in mental illness. Each detailed structure comes with information on functions, disorders, brain damage, case studies, and links to modern research.

(Continued)

Created by Vivid Apps and AXS Biomedical Animation Studio for the Dolan DNA Learning Center (DNALC) at Cold Spring Harbor Laboratory (CSHL). The 3-D brain is derived from the Genes to Cognition (G2C) Online website funded by the Dana Foundation and Hewlett Foundation.

911 Paramedic
http://www.legacygames.com/
download_games/861/
911_paramedic/

This game is set in a big city and provides the player with a variety of interactive elements including simulated patient care, ambulance driving, and communication with the hospital. This 2002 game runs on PC or Mac (OS 8.1). The manufacturer states it is an entertainment-based game, not intended for clinical education.

ACLS Sim Lite iPhone App
http://itunes.apple.com/us/app/
acls-sim-lite/id361156185?mt=8

This App in an Advanced Cardiac Life Support simulator based on the International Consensus on Science published in the Guidelines 2005 for Cardiopulmonary Resuscitation and Emergency Cardiovascular Care. This free version has one clinical scenario named "Sudden collapse at health club."

ACLS Simulator
www.anesoft.com/products/
acls-simulator.aspx

The ACLS Simulator 7 Package incorporates three modules—Rhythm for ECG rhythm recognition, ACLS Simulator for real-time megacode simulation, and writer to help you write your own case scenarios. This easy to use package is based on the most recent American Heart Association algorithms, medications, and dosages. A colorful graphic interface, automated record-keeping, and an on-line help system create a unique and realistic training environment. Interpret the ECG; assess the patient; control the airway, breathing, and circulation; defibrillate; and administer cardiac medications. You must act quickly in this real-time simulation or the patient's condition will deteriorate!

ACLS Simulator iPhone App
http://itunes.apple.com/us/app/
acls-simulator/id360889533?mt=8

This App is an Advanced Cardiac Life Support simulator based on the International Consensus on Science published in the Guidelines 2005 for Cardiopulmonary Resuscitation and Emergency Cardiovascular Care. ACLS SImulator for the iPhone comes with 12 cases.
The first 6 cases cover the Pulseless Arrest Algorithm. Cases 1–3 are ventricular fibrillation, cases 4–5 are pulseless ventricular tachycardia, and case 6 is asystole. The remainder of the cases review the ACLS Tachycardia Algorithm.

(Continued)

AidaOnline 2
www.2aida.net/welcome/

Online & downloadable versions of a game that simulates blood glucose level based on changes in diet and insulin level. Useful for teaching medical students or for the general public.

AnatomyLab
www.AnatomyLab.com

AnatomyLab is an interactive application available for the iPhone and iPod Touch that allows you to follow the dissection process of an actual human body with clear, photographic images. AnatomyLab allows you to progress through many levels of dissection while labeling and studying the different anatomical structure. Labels are accompanied by text describing the structure and function.

ATP3 Lipids
http://atp3lipids.com/ATP3_Lipids.html

ATP3 is a cognitive aid in the form of an iPhone Application designed to assist clinicians in developing cholesterol and lipid management programs for their patients. ATP3 Lipids is developed by Evan Schoenberg, M.D.

Baby CPR
Transcension Healthcare
www.babycpr-app.com/

Baby CPR is a mobile application that includes interactive scenarios and lets you practice the techniques of infant CPR on your mobile device.

Baylor College of Medicine:
Family Eats 2
www.archimage.com/health_games.cfm

Baylor College of Medicine was funded to give the 2004 Family Eats program a face-lift to appeal to today's modern African American mom. A new web environment complete with custom artwork and animated characters. Like its predecessor, Family Eats 2 includes educational animations, custom designed admin tools, and personal tracking for the site visitor. The program aims to address barriers busy families face when trying to plan and prepare healthy meals together.

Baylor College of Medicine:
Squire's Quest! 2
www.archimage.com/health_games.cfm

The Squire's Quest! 2 research project is the follow-up to CNRC's successful Squire's Quest! project. Eight animated characters interact with the player, a Squire, who must save the mediaeval Kingdom of Fivealot from the sneaky King Ssynster by meeting FJV goals and earning enough badges to become a Knight. Squire's Quest! 2 includes over 60 minutes of animation which guides the player through a rich storyline, ten casual games, a virtual kitchen, and FJV behavior-change components.

Biomedicine Research Lab
http://slurl.com/secondlife/
Biomedicine%20Research%20Labs/53/
169/21

Biomedicine Research Lab is the digital headquarters of RL organization S.H.R.O. of Philadelphia, PA. According to their press release S.H.R.O. is committed to excellence in basic genetic research to cure and diagnose

(Continued)

cancer, cardiovascular diseases, diabetes, and other chronic illnesses, and to foster the training of young international doctors in a spirit of professionalism and humanism. Thus far, they have used the virtual location to hold several meetings.

Bioterrorisk
www.uic.edu/sph/prepare/bioterrorisk/

Bioterrorisk is a case-based, mini-course in hazard recognition, interagency communication, risk assessment, and risk communication for the public health workforce.

Blood Typing
http://nobelprize.org/educational/
medicine/landsteiner/landsteiner.html

Match the correct blood with the patients to help keep them alive! This educational game explores the 1930 Nobel Prize in Physiology or Medicine awarded for the discovery of human blood groups made in 1901.

Brain Gain
www.playnormous.com/
game_braingain.cfm

"Brain Gain" is not your average online quiz game! This Playnormous original tests knowledge of food selection, portion size, meal balance, and fruit/vegetable choice in a retro watercolor world. Give your entire brain a workout as Professor Mad Monster grades your reaction time, vocabulary level, math skills, and problem-solving abilities.

Bubble Rubble
www.playnormous.com/
game_bubbletrouble.cfm

"Bubble Trouble" was the first online game created exclusively for Playnormous. Kids and their parents learn to distinguish between different levels of physical activity by helping an underwater monster, Chicken Dawg, collect his aerobic exercise minutes for the day. But be careful, popping strength activity bubbles yield no aerobic minutes, and sedentary activities turn into rocks which block the screen.

Cine-Med Suture Tying Kit
http://cine-med.com/index.
php?nav=assistant&id=SUT100

All-in-one surgical knot and stitch practice kit. Designed for the beginning practitioner to learn, practice, and become proficient with the three knot tying methods and six basic stitches and stitching patterns. Teach yourself how to tie surgical knots and place surgical stitches correctly. Covers fundamentals of square knot placement, knot security, helpful hints, and time-saving tips.
The Model
Contents: patented model designed as a platform to practice knot tying and stitch placement skills, instruments, suture, skin simulator, and tissue pads. The tissue pad and skin simulator are replaceable to allow you to practice as much as needed to become proficient in these techniques.

(Continued)

Suture and Tying Kit Beneficial To: Medical Students, Surgical First Assistants, PA Students, DO Students, Emergency Room Assistants, Veterinary Students, Paramedics, Nurse Practitioners, Military Corpsman

Classical Genetics Simulator
www.cgslab.com/

CGS is a web-based software that allows biology students to apply lessons in Mendelian genetics to real-world scenarios.

CliniSpace™, Innovations in Learning Inc.
www.clinispace.com

CliniSpace™ offers the next generation of training environments for healthcare professionals—immersive, authentic, 3-D virtual environments that replicate the familiar surroundings of daily work.

Combat Medic
www.americasarmy.com/aa/intel/roles.php?id=3

Players can play/assume various military roles including "Combat Medic." This provides situated learning in a VR environment; the role of the Medic is of interest to healthcare educators since players attend a virtual class before treating virtual patients in virtual combat.

Combat Medic Sustainment Training, SimQuest
www.simquest.com/cmst.html

This web-based advanced distributed learning platform helps combat medics maintain their critical thinking and decision making skills in fulfillment of their sustainment training requirements. Users assess and treat casualties within the context of case scenarios based on real-life situations encountered in current conflicts, which enhances performance and increases lifesaving potential.

Comfort Zone: Prostate Cancer Treatment Options
www.archimage.com/health_games.cfm

Comfort Zone is a web-based game, designed for the Abramson Center for the Future of Health. It gives recently diagnosed prostate cancer patients the ability to explore their questions and concerns about treatment options. The game uses friendly spin-the-wheel and card game mechanics, making play easy for older adult audiences. This is coupled with a complex data matrix, backed by baseline patient data and posttreatment surveys. Through gameplay, patients are able to create an informed list of questions for their doctor.

Control of the Cell Cycle
http://nobelprize.org/educational/medicine/2001/cellcycle.html

The game is about the different phases in ordinary cell division, mitosis. Between each phase there are several "checkpoints" to make sure that nothing happened to the genetic material on the way.

Critical Care
www.anesoft.com/products/critical-care-simulator.aspx

The Critical Care Simulator is an exciting real-time graphical simulator that reproduces patient care in an Intensive Care Unit or Emergency Room. Five different critically ill patients are

(Continued)

presented and you must manage the airway, ventilation, fluids, and medications to improve the simulated patient's condition. Optimize the patient's hemodynamic state with vasoactive infusions as guided by invasive monitoring. Many emergency situations will occur requiring rapid diagnosis and proper treatment to avoid disaster. An on-line expert help system is available and an automated record-keeping system provides a detailed chart for the case.

Electrocardiogram
http://nobelprize.org/educational/
medicine/ecg/ecg.html

The Electrocardigram educational game and related readings are based on the 1924 Nobel Prize in Physiology or Medicine, which was awarded for the discovery of the electrocardiogram. Work your way through a number of ECG interpretations.

Escape from Diab
www.archimage.com/diab.cfm

Escape from Diab is a serious videogame adventure in healthy eating and exercise. The project is a production of Archimage, Inc. in collaboration with the Children's Nutrition Research Center of Houston's Baylor College of Medicine on the project. Escape from Diab is funded by a grant from the National Institute of Diabetes and Digestive and Kidney Diseases of the National Institutes of Health. Escape from Diab puts players inside a sci-fi action adventure where healthy lifestyle choices are the keys to winning.

Family Eats 2
www.archimage.com/project.
cfm?id=152&cat=mmedia

Baylor College of Medicine was funded to give the 2004 Family Eats program a face-lift to appeal to today's modern African American mom. Archimage created a brand new web environment complete with custom artwork and animated characters. Like its predecessor, Family Eats 2 includes educational animations, custom designed admin tools, and personal tracking for the site visitor.

Food Fury
www.playnormous.com/game_foodfury.
cfm

"Food Fury" was funded by The Aetna Foundation as part of the Games for Wellness collaborative led by Dr. Cynthia Phelps and the University of Texas Health Science Center. This online game targets 3rd–5th graders to teach and change behavior around food choice and portion control.

Free Dive, BreakAway, Ltd
http://www.breakawaygames.com/
serious-games/solutions/healthcare/

Free Dive is a pediatric pain management game where the user is immersed in a 3-D environment where they can swim with turtles and fish and find hidden treasure. The game is designed to help distract patients who have undergone painful medical treatments.

(Continued)

Heart Murmur Simulation
www.youtube.com/
watch?v=xJY2lwbzop4

The Heart Murmur Simulation gives you a greater understanding of what a heart murmur actually is and the conditions for when it will happen.

HumanSim™, Applied Research Associates - Virtual Heroes
www.humansim.com/

HumanSim™ will enable healthcare professionals to sharpen their assessment and decision making skills without risk to patients in realistic, challenging, immersive environments that are instrumented to provide meaningful performance feedback.

Immune Responses
http://nobelprize.org/educational/
medicine/immuneresponses/game/
index.html

The Immune Responses production is based on several Nobel Prizes in Physiology or Medicine awarded for discoveries related to Immune Responses, from the first Nobel Prize in 1901 until today. Start with going through the 10 interactive stops in the Immune Responses production. Afterward, you can read the overview article "The Immune System: In Defence of our Lives" which provides an in-depth reading about the Nobel Prize–awarded achievements related to the immune system.

Immune System Defender
http://nobelprize.org/educational/
medicine/immunity/game/index.html

In this game, you are a trainee soldier of the Immune System Defense Forces, defending a human against bacterial infection. You have two missions to complete. In the first, you must command a team of white blood cells called granulocytes to fight against bacteria invading the blood system through a finger wound. In the second mission, you must command an army of macrophages and dendritic cells to fight the invading bacteria.

iMurmur
www.phalanxdev.com/

iMurmur is a practical application that teaches you how to recognize and diagnose heart murmurs. The heart sounds are presented in a rapid quiz format and are organized by clinical relevance emphasizing sounds you will encounter most frequently. In addition to a visual diagram of each murmur, you have the option to learn more; you can read about key clinical characteristics, what generates the murmur's unique sound, its pathology, and basic concepts on how to proceed with therapy. iMurmur also includes options to create custom quizzes or to listen to specific murmurs from the collection.

iVCL (Virtual Cath Lab)
http://itunes.apple.com/us/app/ivcl/
id379011867?mt=8

A c-arm simulator and anatomical viewer designed to teach all medical staff and students hand-to-eye coordination skills and anatomical positioning concepts in a radiation-free environment.

(Continued)

Juice Jumble
www.playnormous.com/
game_juicejumble.cfm

Juice Jumble uses online game play to empower kids and their parents to make more informed choices regarding fruit drink selection. Players explore the oftentimes confusing topic of beverage content by chaining drinks that contain 100% fruit juice, only some fruit juice, and no fruit juice.

Lunch Crunch
www.playnormous.com/
game_lunchcrunch.cfm

Lunch Crunch was designed to educate kids and their parents about meal balance and how to effectively use the 5-A-Day plan by adding fruit and vegetables to lunchtime meals. The player must help the lunch line by filling school trays with two fruits or vegetables.

Malaria: Mosquito
http://nobelprize.org/educational/
medicine/malaria/mosquito.html

The Mosquito and Parasite educational games and related reading, are based on the 1902 and 1907 Nobel Prize in Physiology or Medicine. The 1902 Nobel Prize was awarded for the discovery of the parasite causing malaria and for understanding that the Anoheles mosquito was involved in causing malaria. The 1904 Nobel Prize in Physiology or Medicine was awarded for the discovery of the parasite in human blood. Take control of a mosquito and try to find a human to bite and draw blood from! In the mosquito game you stear a mosquito toward humans while you also have to avoid DDT, mosquito nets, buts, and birds to succeed in your mission.

Malaria: Parasite
http://nobelprize.org/educational/
medicine/malaria/parasite.html

Malaria is one of the world's most common diseases, caused by a parasite that is transmitted to humans by a female mosquito's bite. Take control of a parasite, try to find your way inside a human being, and multiply as fast as possible! In the Parasite game you are to guide a parasite through the blood vessels, meantime you must avoid colliding with antibodies and other immune cells. First, guide the parasite to the liver where it could multiply, then guide it to a red blood cell where it can multiply again, before your mission is over. For high score you have to be very skilled with the arrow buttons—it could be quite hard to stear the mosquito and the parasite in these games if you're not used to it.

MOC Breast Disease™ SimQuest
www.simquest.com/moc.html

In this web-based advanced distributed learning platform, surgeons maintain expertise in their area of specialty, enabling them to meet their maintenance of certification (MOC) requirements. Management of virtual patients from initial presentation through imaging requests, diagnostic procedures, and surgical

(Continued)

intervention enables surgeons to maintain cognitive expertise in their area of specialty, thus promoting quality surgical care. The clinical practice addressed here is management of breast disease.

MRI: The Magnetic Miracle
http://nobelprize.org/educational/
medicine/mri/about.html

The MRI educational game is based on the 2003 Nobel Prize in Physiology or Medicine, which was awarded for discoveries concerning MRI— magnetic resonance imaging, a technique making it possible to get images of soft tissue inside the body. Assist in MRI procedures and sorting images.

MyBody
www.anatomylab.com/iphone/

MyBody is an iPhone and iPod Touch application designed with the general public in mind. It provides the user with an interactive virtual cadaver dissection. The software is based from real cadavers, skeletons, and historical specimens.

My Pyramid Blast Off
http://teamnutrition.usda.gov/resources/
game/blastoff_game.html#

My Pyramid Blast Off is an interactive game for kids, developed by the USDA. It educates the players about health food choices. The goal is to fill the shoot with enough healthy food for one day without overloading the fuel tank.

Nanoswarm: Invasion from Inner Space
www.nanoswarmthegame.com/

Nanoswarm is a role-playing PC adventure game, funded by the NIH, which is designed to target obesity and type 2 diabetes in children. Nanoswarm is the story of four teenage scientists and the player, nicknamed Wings, who must save the world from a plague that threatens the health of the global community. They also pilot a microscopic ship through the body of Fred, their friend who suddenly became ill from an unknown condition that threatens the health of the world. As Wings, the player must set and achieve real-life goals to eat more fruit and vegetables and be physically active to win the game.

Netter's Anatomy for iPhone and iPod Touch
www.modalitylearning.com/
netters-anatomy.asp

Netter's Anatomy by Modality Inc. allows you to navigate through images with the flick of a finger, pinch to zoom, and tap to test your knowledge of muscles, bones, vessels, viscera joints, and more. Use study mode to explore images at your own pace and quiz mode to test yourself on what you know.

Neurological Eye Simulator
http://cim.ucdavis.edu/eyes/eyesim.htm

From UC-Davis Health System/School of Medicine: "This application simulates eye motion and demonstrates the effects of disabling one or more of the 12 eye muscles and one or more of the 6 cranial nerves that

(Continued)

control eye motion. The purpose of this simulator is to teach medical students and doctors how the eye motion will change with pathology of the eye muscles and cranial nerves and what to look for during a standard neurological eye exam."

Pandemic Response™ SimQuest
www.simquest.com/pandemic.html

In this PC-based virtual tabletop exercise, users train for, experiment with, and experience the realities of a pandemic influenza outbreak in the context of a treatment hospital. Playing the role of a hospital administrator, you'll need to manage staff, resources, public relations, safety, and financials in an effort to keep your facility operational as a pandemic flu event is about to deliver a super surge of patients to your doorstep.

Your advanced strategic planning and tactical decision making will be tested as you lead your facility through the crisis.

Practice responding to an infectious disease outbreak will improve preparedness, both from the patient management and incident command standpoints, and could be instrumental in mitigating the spread and effects of disease. We are seeking beta site partners for Pandemic Response; please contact us for more information.

Perfect OB Wheel
http://perfectobwheel.com/
Perfect_OB_Wheel/Perfect_OB_Wheel.
html

Perfect OB Wheel is a pregnancy wheel available for the iPhone, iPod Touch, and the Windows Phone 7. Perfect OB Wheel is a downloadable app which provides the user with a number of estimated benchmarks including: Estimated Due Date, LMP Date, Conception Date, 1st Trimester End Date, 2nd Trimester End Date, and Current Gestational Age, Current Conceptional Age, and Expected Fetal Length based on standard fetal growth curves. Perfect OB Wheel was developed by Evan Schoenberg, M.D.

**Prevention Communication
Research Database**
www.health.gov/communication

The Prevention Communication Research Database (PCRD), a project of the Office of Disease Prevention and Health Promotion (ODPHP), Department of Health and Human Services (HHS), is a searchable collection of audience research conducted or sponsored by HHS agencies.

Pulse!! BreakAway, Ltd
www.breakawaygames.com/
serious-games/solutions/healthcare/

Pulse!! is a virtual clinic learning lab for healthcare professionals. It is designed for military medical personnel to practice clinical

(Continued)

skills to help in the response of injuries during catastrophic incidents.

Pyramid Pile Up Plus
www.playnormous.com/
game_food_pyramid.cfm

Playnormous Pyramid Pile Up Plus is a strategy nutrition game designed to teach you all about the food groups. Learn what foods go in which categories, the benefits of whole grain and low fat, and what discretionary calories are.

Rapid Trauma Training Systems™ SimQuest
www.simquest.com/rts.html

In this simulation/strategy case-management system, player surgeons apply trauma decision making skills in the context of a forward surgical team (FST).

Surgeons are presented with real-world combat case scenarios that they manage virtually. Each scenario is based on an actual case from recent conflicts and users work within the resource-constrained environment typical of an FST.

Enhanced predeployment training of U.S. military surgeons in the essential skills of trauma surgery within a combat environment has the very real potential to improve patient outcomes.

Real Anatomy
http://anatomylab.com/iphone/demo.htm

Real Anatomy is a comprehensive software program based on cadaver dissection. The program includes over 600,000 images that can be imported into other programs like PowerPoint presentations. Includes audio pronunciation of structures and provides users with multiple testing modes.

RespiTrainer® Advance
www.ingmarmed.com/respi_advance.htm

This airway management and ventilation task trainer gives the essential features of a high-end respiratory mannikin plus true ventilation data.

RealCare Shaken Baby
www.realityworks.com/
infantsimulations/shakenbaby.asp

Just one thoughtless shake can cause permanent brain damage or death. This simulation begins with the cries of an inconsolable infant. Accelerometers inside the head measure the force on the brain when shaken. LED lights show the damage to specific areas of the brain in real time. The simulator's cries stop abruptly for all the wrong reasons. The Shaken Baby Syndrome Simulator comes with a curriculum.

Simquest
http://simquest.com/

SimQuest develops advanced biomedical simulators, serious games, and advanced distributed learning applications for medical training, and is involved with injury database development/analysis. The company's goal is to provide healthcare professionals with tools to enable them to develop and perfect their skills without risk to patients.

(Continued)

SonoMan System
www.simulab.com/product/
ultrasound-trainers/sonoman-system

The SonoMan System provides a platform for teaching students how to read diagnostic ultrasound imaging. The system includes a soft tissue body form with internal and external landmarks and a simulated probe.

Speed Anatomy, Speed Bones MD, Speed Angiography MD, Speed Muscles MD
http://speedanatomy.com/

This is a series of anatomy games for the iPhone, iPod Touch, iPad, and Android designed by Benoid Essiambre. The Speed Anatomy games are fun and addictive games that test your speed and challenge your memory.

Squires Quest II
www.archimage.com/project.
cfm?id=150&cat=mmedia

The Squire's Quest! 2 research project is the second iteration of the Children's Nutrition Research Center's highly acclaimed multimedia program Squire's Quest!, which was clinically proven to increase fruit, juice, and vegetable consumption in elementary school children by one serving size. Eight animated characters interact with the player, a Squire, who must save the mediaeval Kingdom of Fivealot from the sneaky King Ssynster by meeting FJV goals and earning enough badges to become a Knight. Squire's Quest! 2 includes over 60 minutes of cut scenes which guide the player through rich storyline, ten casual games, a virtual kitchen, and FJV behavior-change components. SQ!2 was created for Dr. Debbe Thompson of the USDA/ARS Children's Nutrition Research Center at Baylor College of Medicine.

StereoVision
www.meleritmedical.com/html/pdf/
new/MeleritStereoVision.pdf

Melerit StereoVision gives the user a stereoscopic view of 3-D objects in a computer-generated world. It gives the user a feeling of looking at a real object through a stereo microscope. Some examples of typical uses includes eye surgery, spine surgery, biological, chemistry, and forensic studies.

SurgicalSIM Cholecystectomy
www.meti.com/
products_ss_cholecystectomy.htm

SurgicalSIM VR is a multispecialty, multimodality surgical training system that combines psychomotor skills training and assessment with didactic content to support surgical education. The Cholecystectomy Learning Module focuses on training in the removal of the gallbladder with minimal risk of injury to the bile ducts and the surrounding structures.

Teen Choice
www.illusionstudioinc.com/
project_TeenChoice_EatBreakfast.
html?proj=Teenchoice_EatBreakfast&i

Teen Choice is a web-based project focusing on the barriers teens face when trying to eat healthy and be physically active. Our studio was hired to produce 12 computer-animated shorts to act as role model stories for the project. This was a collaboration with Illusion Studio, Archimage, and Baylor College.

(Continued)

The Ear Pages
http://nobelprize.org/educational/
medicine/ear/game/index.html

The Ear Pages, consisting of readings, animations, and quizzes is based on the 1961 Nobel Prize in Physiology or Medicine, which was awarded for the discovery of how sound is analyzed and communicated in the cochlea in the inner ear. You can choose between three levels of quizzes: beginner, advanced, and expert. If you manage to get all the answers correct you will appear on the "High score of the week" list!

The Split Brain Experiments
http://nobelprize.org/educational/
medicine/split-brain/splitbrainexp.html

The Split Brain Experiments game and related reading are based on the 1981 Nobel Prize in Physiology or Medicine, which was awarded for discoveries concerning differences in the right and left brain hemispheres. In this game you perform the classic split brain experiment used by Nobel Laureate Roger Sperry when he discovered differences between the right and left hemispheres of the brain. See how the patient reacts and try to figure out why he is acting the way he does. In order to be able to proceed with your research you have to get more money, and when applying for more grants you have to report on your findings. If you manage to make correct conclusions you'll be awarded with more grants and eventually your research will be published in a scientific journal.

Virtual Bacterial Identification Lab
www.hhmi.org/biointeractive/vlabs/
bacterial_id/index.html

The purpose of Virtual Bacterial Identification Lab is to familiarize you with the science and techniques used to identify different types of bacteria based on their DNA sequence. Not long ago, DNA sequencing was a time-consuming, tedious process. With readily available commercial equipment and kits, it is now routine. The techniques used in this lab are applicable in a wide variety of settings, including scientific research and forensic labs.

Virtual Cardiology Lab
www.hhmi.org/biointeractive/vlabs/
cardiology/

The focus of the Virtual Cardiology Lab is on heritable diseases of the heart. You are cast here as a virtual intern to accompany a doctor examining three different patients. Each patient is examined, using more than one diagnostic tool, and at each stage, the doctor will invite you to examine the patient yourself and ask for your opinion.

Virtual Immunology Lab
www.hhmi.org/biointeractive/vlabs/
immunology/index.html

This virtual laboratory will demonstrate how such a test, termed an enzyme-linked immunosorbent assay (ELISA), is carried out and some of the key experimental problems that may be encountered. Students will learn

(Continued)

about the assay procedure and the equipment and materials that are needed. By completing this exercise, students will gain a better understanding of experimental design, key concepts in immunological reactions, and interpretation of data.

Virtual Iraq
www.virtuallybetter.com/IraqOverview.html

"Virtual Iraq" has a virtual reality environment suitable for therapy of anxiety disorders resulting from the high-stress environment. The treatment involves exposing the patient to a virtual environment containing the feared situation rather than taking the patient into the actual environment or having the patient imagine the stimulus. Not available for purchase by the public.

Virtual Neurophysiology Lab
www.hhmi.org/biointeractive/vlabs/neurophysiology/index.html

In the Virtual Neurophysiology Lab you will record electrical activities of individual neurons while you deliver mechanical stimulus to the attached skin. Inject florescent dyes into the neurons to visualize their morphology. Identify the neurons based on the morphology and the response to stimuli, comparing them to previously published results.

Virtual Patient
http://ict.usc.edu/projects/virtual_patient/C40

Virtual Patients are advanced conversational virtual human agents that have been applied to the psychiatric medical field. These interactive agents portray a patient with a clinical or physical condition and can interact verbally and nonverbally with a clinician in an effort to teach interpersonal skills.

This project focuses on making believable, interpretable, and responsive virtual humans that deviate from the norm and express both rational and irrational behaviors. (Other groups typically focus on developing rational virtual humans that mimic rationality.)

This is a University of Southern California Institute for Creative Technologies project (http://ict.usc.edu/).

Virtual Transgenic Fly Lab
www.hhmi.org/biointeractive/vlabs/transgenic_fly/index.html

The lab will familiarize you with the science and techniques used to make transgenic flies. Transgenic organisms, which contain DNA that is inserted experimentally, are used to study many biological processes. In this lab, you will create a transgenic fly to study circadian rhythms. The fly glows only when a certain gene involved in circadian rhythms is activated. After making the glowing fly, you will use it to explore basic principles of circadian biology and genetics.

MAJOR SIMULATOR COMPANIES

CAE Healthcare (formally METI)
http://caehealthcare.com

METI/CAE has expertise and focuses on mannikin-based simulators and related products to facilitate the simulation-based education.

Laerdal
www.laerdal.com/Simulation

Laerdal has expertise and focuses on mannikin-based simulators and related products to facilitate the simulation-based education.

Gaumard
www.gaumard.com/

Gaumard has expertise and focuses on mannikin-based simulators and related products to facilitate the simulation-based education.

Glossary

Adragogy: Of or pertaining to adult education (Merriam & Caffarella, 2007).

Appeal: Appeal refers to the capacity in which a learning strategy can keep learners' attention and engagement. Appeal is commonly associated with the visual look and feel or cognitive challenge associated with a virtual environment or game-based learning. However, it also refers to usability or ease of use of the environment or game.

Augmented reality: Augmented reality supplements the *real-world* such that actual objects existing in the *real-world* appear to coexist with virtual objects, computer-generated images that are representations of actual objects (Azuma et al., 2001).

Avatar: The term avatar is originally from Greek mythology. The gods would take the shape of mortals in the form of human avatars to walk the earth. In video games and virtual environments, an avatar transcends two planes of existence: the real world and the in-world or virtual world. The avatar or player-character is the embodiment of the person playing the game. Players live in and interact with the virtual or game-based environment through their avatars. Contemporary game-based and virtual reality avatars are often highly malleable and can be customized by individual players. Some will relate the avatar to a player's in-world alter ego (Bauman, 2010, p. 183).

Badges: Badges serve as a validated indicator of success and provide a tangible record of achievement. Badges make individuals' accomplishments visible for others to see whether they are provided within the virtual or the real-world. From the historical nursing example, the number of stripes presented on the classic nurse's cap denoted the amount and level of training a student nurse had accomplished. Badges play an important role in supporting participation within communities, encouraging learning, and developing identity and reputation (http://www.dmlcompetition.net).

Blog(s): Lightweight content management and publishing system comprised of posts (i.e., regularly updated content, usually arranged chronologically), pages (similar to traditional webpages) and media. Can be personal or collaborative and often can contain opinions, news, media, scholarly information, and more.

Bot: The term bot originated from early work related to artificial intelligence. It can be used for any automated software agent that behaves in an artificially autonomous manner. Bots were often used as early versions of nonplayer characters in text-based virtual worlds. The term bot also includes agents such as web browser spider bots and Internet Relay Chat Bots (IRC Bot), commonly referred to as chat bots. Spider bots mine web pages to collect and analyze data, while chat bots simulate conversations with game players (Bauman, 2010, p. 185).

CLAS standards: National Standards for Culturally and Linguistically Appropriate Services in Health Care (U.S. Department of Health and Human Services).

Controlled vocabulary: A set of standardized terms used to precisely describe a concept or domain. Controlled vocabulary focuses more on the words than the ideas, and helps disambiguate and clarify synonyms, alternate spellings, and so on.

Created environment: An environment that has been specifically engineered to replicate an actual existing environment, producing sufficient authenticity and environmental fidelity to allow for the suspension of disbelief. Simulated environments, whether fixed in the case of mannikin-based simulation laboratories, or existing in virtual reality, are created environments (Bauman, 2007; Bauman, 2010, p. 185).

Crosswalking or crosswalk: Taking different systems and mapping out which elements in one are found in another. Allows for automated search across systems that use different terms for the same concepts. UMLS is an example of crosswalking different thesauri into one system.

Dashboard: Computer interface with many related functions packed into a small space (as in an airplane cockpit or high-end automobile).

Designed experience: A designed experience is engineered to include structured activities targeted to facilitate interactions that drive anticipated experiences. In other words, the experience embodies structured activity and the environment in which the activities take place. Many theme parks are based in part on the theory of designed experience (Bauman, 2010, p. 185; Squire, 2006).

Digital immigrant: Refers to those of us who have adopted digital technology as adults or later in life. Not all digital immigrants were born prior to the widespread adoption of digital media and devices. The concept of the digital immigrant may not always map to a generational context and can relate to people just encountering innovative digital technology (Presnsky, 201).

Digital native: Generally referring to those people who have always been part of the net (as in Internet) or digital generation. Digital natives are fluent in the language of the digital environment. They possess an innate sense of media literacy (Prensky, 2001).

Easter egg: Novel facets of virtual reality and game-based environments that provide useful information, tangible reward, or entertainment value of some kind. They are often integrated into environments to provide just-in-time information and to promote a sense of environmental exploration (Bauman, 2010, p. 185).

Effectiveness: The effectiveness of an instructional strategy is measured in relation to the goals and objectives of the instruction (Reigeluth & Merrill, 1979), and the accuracy, comprehensiveness, and freshness of the content (Weston, McAlpine, & Bordonaro, 1995).

Efficiency: Efficiency, in the context of education refers to the design, development, and delivery of instruction "in ways that use the least resources for the same or better results" (Januszewski & Molenda, 2008, p. 59).

E-learning: In general, e-learning refers to any type of instruction that takes place through the Internet (Pastore, 2002). In other words, it refers to any instruction that occurs via any online application such as video-conferencing tools, web browsers, virtual world applications, and so on.

Environmental fidelity: Relates to the physical surroundings or representation of physical surroundings in which a simulation or game takes place; in other words, the theatrics. If the theatrics are sufficiently accurate, players or learners are more likely to become immersed in the learning experience (Bauman, 2007; Gaba, 2004). Environmental fidelity drives psychological fidelity.

Evidence-centered design (ECD): An assessment framework grounded in evidentiary reasoning. It has two main components: the conceptual assessment framework and the four-process delivery model.

External validity: The degree to which the results of a given study or experiment can be generalized to settings or populations other than the ones studied. This is particularly salient when using created environments to conduct research (Polit & Hungler, 1999). When assessing external validity one asks, "Can the results occurring in a simulated or digital environment be generalized to actual practice?"

Facebook: A popular social media website. From the context of this textbook it is an example of one of the tools associated with Web 2.0 discussion.

Folksonomy: An informal, bottom-up way of organizing information for later use. Contrasted with taxonomy, which is more formal and top-down, and is usually done for professional or standards-based uses.

Game-based platform: An environment that provides a narrative and system of rewards for accomplishing specific tasks and objectives. Game-based platforms use virtual environments to stage the game. Not all virtual reality environments are game-based (Bauman, 2010, p. 186).

Haptic: Refers to tactile touch sensation. In virtual reality and game-based environments, it specifically refers to the touch sensation feedback that the learner or player receives from the game or environment. In console-based video games, haptic feedback often occurs through vibrations in the hand-held game controller (Bauman, 2010, p. 186).

Heads-up display (HUD): Any transparent display that presents data without requiring users to look away from their usual viewpoints.

High-fidelity: A level of sophistication often achieved through sophisticated computer modeling that allows students engaging simulators and *created environments* to explore complex multidimensional skills. *High-fidelity* simulators and environments provide ongoing and immediate feedback as learning experiences progress (Bauman, 2007; Lane, Slavin, & Ziv, 2001).

Hypothesis: A prediction of expected outcome and includes a statement of outcome as it relates to the variables being investigated. It is the predicted answer to the research question (Polit & Hungler, 1999).

Information technology (IT): The acquisition, processing, storage, and use of information (in any format) by computers and telecommunications technology.

In situ: Learning that takes place in an actual clinical environment. In situ simulation places simulation-based technology in the real world to facilitate authentic clinical learning experiences.

Institutional Review Board (IRB): A group of individuals, but generally a formal committee from an institution that reviews the ethical considerations of proposed research and grants approval for the research projects to proceed. From an educational perspective the ethical considerations most often relate to the ethical treatment of human subjects (Polit & Hungler, 1999).

Instructional design (ID): The practice of implementing pedagogy using a systemic approach that is effective and efficient for teachers while being appealing to learners. Often used with online and new media sources, but can refer to any form of instruction or other learning experiences.

Interface: The tool that allows a user to interact with the electronic medium, software, or tool. See also *Dashboard*.

Internal validity: The degree that the researcher can attribute or infer that outcome of an experimental treatment or independent variable is responsible for observed effect or behavior (Polit & Hungler, 1999).

In-world: Refers to the game or virtual reality environment. Interactions that are taking place in-world are occurring within the confines of the game or virtual environment (Bauman, 2010, p. 186).

Low-fidelity: Simple and uncomplicated, often demonstrating a concept. Low-fidelity simulators and simulations and environments as less interactive and responsive than their *high-fidelity* counterparts and allow students to explore basic-level unidimensional skills.

Massively multiplayer online games (MMOGs): Video games that are designed to support hundreds of thousands of players simultaneously. MMOGs generally provide at least one constant environment and by necessity are played on the Internet (online). Although many MMOGs are designed to be played using personal computers, many console-based video games also have MMOG capability. MMOGs are sometimes referred to as MOGs (multiplayer online games) (Bauman, 2010, p. 186).

MUVE: Multiuser virtual environments. MUVEs can be accessed through the Internet, allowing users to create an identity and interact with other users in a virtual world in real time.

Nonplayer character: In-world agents of and from the game or virtual environment. NPCs are a function of programming and do not exist outside of the game or virtual environment. NPCs are in-world characters that the players' (learners') avatars interact with. This term originated from paper-based role-playing games like Dungeons and Dragons. It is a narrower definition than bot; however, there is often a blurring between the definitions of bot and NPC (Bauman, 2010, p. 186).

Ontology: A shared vocabulary to describe objects, their properties, and their interrelationships in a domain or field. More simply put, ontologies represent domain-specific knowledge in a structured and consistent fashion to facilitate the organization, sharing, and automated processing of information.

Partial task trainers: Sometimes generically referred to as task trainers, they are simulators that replicate only a portion of a complete process (Cooper & Taqueti, 2004). They often are designed to allow learners to replicate a discrete task using them. They can be of varying levels of fidelity. An example of a partial task trainer is an IV arm or an airway task trainer.

Player character: See *Avatar*.

Power analysis: A technique used in quantitative research to determine the likelihood for the occurrence of a Type II error (concluding that there is no relationship when in fact one does exist). A power analysis used to establish sample size (Polit & Hungler, 1999).

Projective identity: The hybrid identity synthesized from the player's real-world identity and in-world identity. It is the identity that the player adopts within the context of the virtual or game world. The projective identity represents a reconciliation of the player's in-world and real-world experiences (Bauman, 2010, p. 186; Games & Bauman, 2011; Gee, 2003).

Psychological fidelity: Represents a participant's ability to suspend their disbelief in reality and become immersed in the situation. In this way, a virtual experience taking place during a designed experience becomes situated (Bauman, 2007; Gee, 2003).

Qualitative research: A research method focusing on the investigation of phenomena using in-depth analysis of nonnumeric data such as narrative. Qualitative research designs are often flexible and focus on multiple interpretations of data focusing on identified themes. Examples of qualitative research methodologies include but are not limited to grounded theory, phenomenology, and critical theory (Diekelmann, 2003; Polit & Hungler, 1999).

Quantitative research: A research method focusing on the investigation of phenomena using numeric quantification and measurement. There are various types and levels of rigor associated with quantitative research design ranging from observational and descriptive design (less rigorous) and quasi-experimental and experimental design (more rigorous) (Polit & Hungler, 1999).

Real world: Refers to the environment that we live in, not the game or virtual world. One often contrasts in-world experiences with real-world experiences (Bauman, 2010, p. 186).

Research question: A query or question that is specific to the problem statement (Polit & Hungler, 1999).

Resource discovery tools: Tools that facilitate finding desired resources, usually online and digital. "Resource" is used to allow and account for multiple sources of information—books, journal articles, websites, media, and so on. These tools include databases, search engines, library card catalogs, and so on.

Second Life®: A popular proprietary online 3-D virtual reality world created by Linden Lab® where users can socialize, connect, and create using free voice and text chat (www.secondlife.com and www.lindenlab.com).

Serious game: A game that is used to convey objectives found in an academic or institutional curriculum whether or not the initial design elements of the game were intended for the purposes of entertainment or education.

StarCraft 2: A popular real-time strategy game developed by Blizzard Entertainment. There is a strong and growing tournament/competitive culture associated with *StarCraft 2*.

Stealth assessment: Valerie Shute's embedded assessment framework in which evidence-centered design is applied to digital environments (especially games) (Shute, 2011).

Suspension of disbelief: The product of adequate environmental and psychological fidelity. It encompasses or relates to the learner or students' state of mind and allows the student to achieve emotional buy-in during immersion in simulation and game-based experiences.

Tagging: The act of assigning keywords or phrases to content such as journal articles and websites to help organize these resources for later use.

Taxonomy: A structured, hierarchical information classification scheme. Taxonomy is more structured and rigorous than a controlled vocabulary, less descriptive, and more complete than an ontology.

Theatrics: The combination of variables and effects that help to promote *suspension of disbelief.*

Threat assessment: An evaluation used to identify variables that impede day-to-day and crisis management processes.

Twitter: Twitter is a popular social media website. From the context of this textbook it is an example of one of the tools associated with Web 2.0 discussion.

Uncanny valley: A phenomenon that occurs when animated or robotic characters approach life-like fidelity, but fail to allow the viewer to achieve complete suspension of disbelief. The characters can illicit negative emotions and responses from those interacting or viewing them (Mori, 1970).

Unified medical language system (UMLS): UMLS is a metathesaurus (e.g., a thesaurus derived from other thesauruses) that pulls together many different sources in nursing and other health sciences to allow information organization, search, and retrieval. It would, for example, allow searching across disparate databases from one interface.

Virtual patients (VPs): Virtual patients are created using software to replicate authentic nonplayer characters for virtual environments.

Virtual worlds: An environment that hosts a synchronous digital environment, persistent network of people, represented as avatars, facilitated by networked computers (Bell, 2008).

Walkthrough: A form of in-world tutorial that allows players to orient themselves to the virtual or game-based environment. Walkthroughs can be self-guided or can be guided by NPCs and other PCs.

Web 2.0: In general refers to web-based applications that facilitate user-generated content and sharing of that content.

Wiki(s): A wiki is a collaborative tool that predates blogs and is primarily or exclusively text based. It allows for collaborative creation and editing of documents, which makes it a popular tool for academics, and it has some features (like versioning and access control) found in blogs and more complex tools. Wikipedia is a canonical example.

REFERENCES

Azuma, R. T., Baillot, Y., Behringer, R., Feiner, S., Julier, S., & MacIntrye, B. (2001). Recent advances in augmented reality. *IEEE Computer Graphics and Applications*, *21*(6), 34–37.

Bauman, E. (2007). *High fidelity simulation in healthcare*. PhD dissertation, The University of Wisconsin – Madison, United States. Dissertations & Theses @ CIC Institutions database. (Publication no. AAT 3294196 ISBN: 9780549383109 ProQuest document ID: 1453230861).

Bauman, E. (2010). Virtual reality and game-based clinical education. In Gaberson, K. B., & Oermann, M. H. (Eds.), *Clinical teaching strategies in nursing education* (3rd ed.). New York: Springer Publishing Company.

Bell, M. (2008). Toward a definition of virtual worlds. *Journal of Virtual Worlds Research*, *1*(1), 1–5.

Cooper, J. B., & Taqueti, V. R. (2004). A brief history of the development of mannequin simulators for clinical education and training. *Quality and Safety in Health Care*, *13*(Suppl. 1), i11–i18.

Diekelmann, N. L. (Ed.) (2003). *Teaching the practitioners of care: New pedagogies for the health professions*. Madison, WI: The University of Wisconsin Press.

Gaba, D. M. (2004). The future vision of simulation in health care. *Quality and Safety in Health Care*, *13*(Suppl. 1), i2–i10.

Games, I., & Bauman, E. (2011) Virtual worlds: An environment for cultural sensitivity education in the health sciences. *International Journal of Web Based Communities* *7*(2), 187–205.

Gee, J. P. (2003). *What videogames have to teach us about learning and literacy*. New York, NY: Palgrave-McMillan.

Januszewski, A., & Molenda, M. (2008). *Educational technology: A definition with commentary*. New York: Lawrence Erlbaum Associates.

Lane, J. L., Slavin, S., & Ziv, A. (2001). Simulation in medical education: A review. *Simulation & Gaming*, *32*(3), 297–314.

Merriam, S. B., & Caffarella, R. S. (2007). *Learning in adulthood: A comprehensive guide* (3rd ed.). San Francisco, CA: Jossey-Bass.

Mori, M. (1970). The uncanny valley. *Energy*, *7*(4), 33–35.

Pastore, R. (2002). E-learning in education: An overview. *Society for Information Technology and Teacher Education International Conference (SITE)*, *1*, 275–276.

Polit, D. F., & Hungler, B. P. (1999). *Nursing research: Principles and methods* (6th ed.). Philadelphia: Lippincott.

Prensky, M. (2001). Digital natives, digital immigrants. *On the Horizon*, *9*(5), 1–6.

Reigeluth, C. M., & Merrill, M. D. (1979). Classes of instructional variables. *Educational Technology, 29*(3), 5-24.

Shute, V. J. (2011). Stealth assessment in computer-based games to support learning. In Tobias, S., & Fletcher, J. D. (Eds.), *Computer games and instruction.* Charlotte, NC: Information Age Publishers.

Squire, K. (2006). From content to context: Videogames as designed experience. *Educational Researcher, 35*(8), 19-29.

U.S. Department of Health, Human Services. National Standards for Culturally, Linguistically Appropriate Services (CLAS) in Health Care. *Office of Minority Health Resource Center* Retrieved September 15, 2011, from http://www.omhrc.gov/CLAS

Weston, C., McAlpine, L., & Bordonaro, T. (1995). A model for understanding formative evaluation in instructional design. *Educational Technology Research and Development, 43*(3), 29-49.

Index